Chair Yoga Revolution for Seniors Over 60

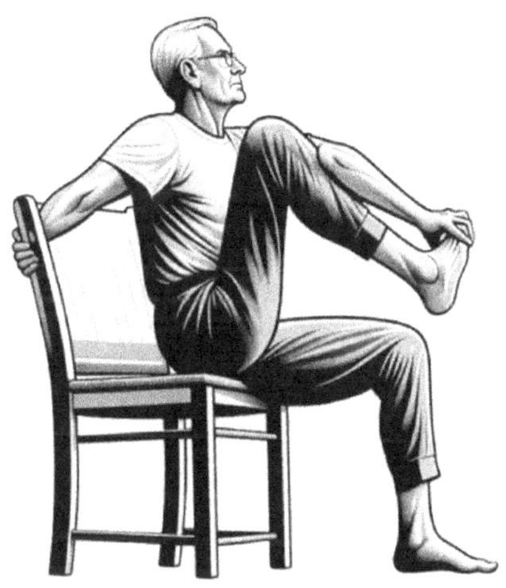

Boost Strength, Flexibility, and Inner Peace: Over 40 Easy-to-Follow Poses and Sequences for Improved Balance, Mobility, and Weight Loss, Illustrated Edition

Clara Harper

1

Table of content

INTRODUCTION...5

The Benefits of Chair Yoga for Seniors...................................8

How to Use This Book 10

Understanding Chair Yoga 12

Setting Up Your Space 14

Safety First: Guidelines for Practicing Chair Yoga 16

Chapter Two: The Exercises 19

   1. Seated Marching 20

   2. Chair Cat-Cow Stretch 22

   3. Seated Mountain Pose (Tadasana) 24

   4. Seated Forward Bend (Paschimottanasana)................26

   5. Chair Pigeon Pose 28

   6. Seated Spinal Twist 30

   7. Seated Side Stretch 32

   8. Wrist and Finger Stretches...34

   9. Ankle Circles...36

   10. Leg Extensions...38

   11. Arm Circles..40

   12. Shoulder Shrugs...42

   13. Neck Stretch..44

   14. Upper Body Twist...46

   15. Toe Taps..48

   16. Heel Raises..50

17. Seated Leg Lifts 52

18. Seated Knee Lifts with a Twist 54

19. Chair Supported Squat.................................56

20. Seated "T" Pose..58

21. Seated Bicycle Crunches 60

22. Arm and Leg Lifts 62

23. Wrist Flexor and Extensor Stretches.........64

24. Shoulder Blade Pinches...............................66

25. Seated Side Bends.......................................68

26. Seated Hamstring Stretch 70

27. Calf Stretches 72

28. Seated Figure Four Stretch 74

29. Neck Rotations 76

30. Seated Ankle Flexion and Extension 78

31. Upper Back and Shoulder Stretch...............80

32. Toe Spread and Squeeze.............................82

33. Seated Hip Circles 84

34. Elbow Circles...86

35. Seated Torso Twists 88

36. Chair Push-Ups..90

17. Seated Knee Extensions 92

38. Hand Clench and Release...........................94

39. Seated Calf Raises 96

40. Breathing Exercises.....................................98

21 Days - challenge 100

Conclusion 103

INTRODUCTION

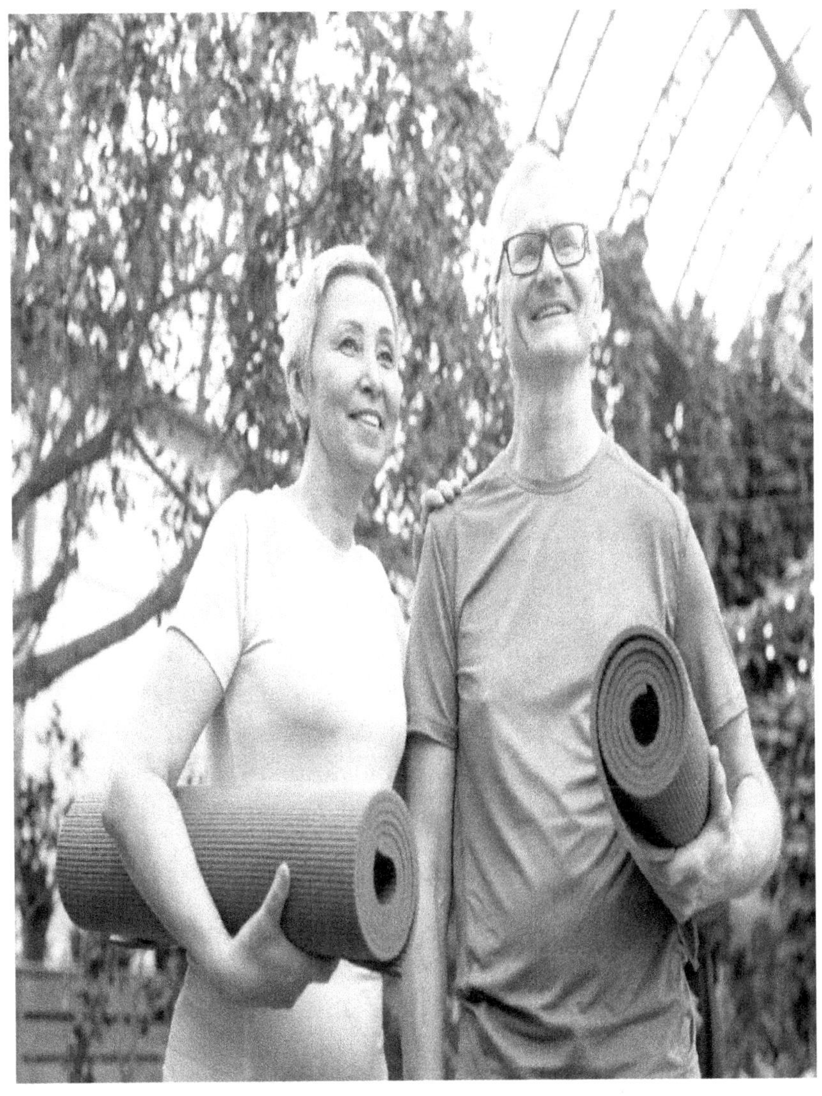

Welcome to a journey that redefines the essence of Yoga, especially for those of us who have crossed into the golden years of over 60. When the mainstream narrative of Yoga often showcases the young and agile, effortlessly folding into poses that seem as much art as exercise, it's easy to feel sidelined. But Yoga, in its truest form, transcends age, flexibility, and every physical boundary we might perceive.

This ancient practice, with roots stretching back over 5,000 years, has always been about adaptation, growth, and the deep connection between mind, body, and spirit. It's a misconception that to reap Yoga's benefits, one must twist into complex shapes or balance precariously on one limb. The truth is far more inclusive and accessible. Chair Yoga, a gentle yet profoundly effective adaptation, stands as a testament to Yoga's versatility, offering the same holistic benefits from the comfort of a chair.

Designed with seniors in mind, Chair Yoga makes the comprehensive benefits of traditional Yoga accessible to everyone, including those who might not feel at home on a traditional yoga mat due to age, mobility issues, or health concerns. It proves that the transformative power of Yoga can be fully experienced without the need for floor-based exercises, making it an ideal practice for enhancing flexibility, strength, balance, and mental clarity, all while seated. This book is an invitation to explore Chair Yoga as a pathway to wellness, tailored specifically for seniors over 60. It's for those who believe that age should not be a barrier to experiencing the joy and multitude of benefits that Yoga offers.

Whether you're encountering Yoga for the first time or looking to adapt your existing practice to suit your current needs, this guide is designed to walk you through every aspect of Chair Yoga. From understanding its foundation to learning how to perform various poses and sequences, this book aims to equip you with everything you need to embark on a fulfilling Chair Yoga journey.

Chair Yoga is more than just an exercise form; it's a celebration of what our bodies can do, a rediscovery of movement and breath, and a reaffirmation of our capacity to grow and adapt at any age. If you've picked up this book, it's a sign that you're ready to explore new possibilities, to embrace a form of Yoga that acknowledges where you are today and helps you move toward where you want to be tomorrow. Let this be the beginning of a beautiful journey towards health, wellness, and the joy of movement, one chair pose at a time. Let's begin this journey together.

The Benefits of Chair Yoga for Seniors

Chair Yoga, as an accessible and gentle form of Yoga, holds a treasure trove of benefits for seniors, a group for whom mobility, balance, and flexibility may present challenges. This specialized practice adapts the traditional yoga poses to a seated format, making it an inclusive exercise that can be performed anywhere you have access to a chair. Here are the key benefits that Chair Yoga offers to seniors:

Enhanced Flexibility and Mobility: Regular practice gently stretches and strengthens the body, enhancing flexibility and range of motion. This can make daily activities easier and more enjoyable.

Improved Strength and Balance: By engaging various muscle groups, chair yoga helps build strength, which is crucial for maintaining balance and preventing falls—a common concern for seniors.

Stress Reduction and Mental Clarity: The meditative aspects of chair yoga, combined with deep breathing exercises, can significantly reduce stress, anxiety, and depression, promoting mental clarity and a sense of calm.

Better Joint Health and Pain Management: Chair yoga can alleviate pain and improve joint health by gently moving and strengthening areas around the knees, shoulders, hips, and spine.

Enhanced Circulation: The movements in chair yoga help improve blood circulation, which is beneficial for heart health and can aid in reducing swelling and pain in the lower limbs.

Social Interaction and Community: Participating in chair yoga classes can provide a sense of community and reduce feelings of isolation, which is especially important for seniors.

Increased Energy and Alertness: Regular engagement in chair yoga can boost energy levels and contribute to a greater sense of alertness and well-being.

How to Use This Book

This book is designed as a comprehensive guide to introduce you to the practice of Chair Yoga, ensuring that you can safely and effectively incorporate it into your life. Here's how to get the most out of this resource:

Start with the Introduction: Familiarize yourself with what chair yoga is and why it is particularly beneficial for seniors. This will give you a good foundation and understanding of the practice.

Progress at Your Own Pace: Each chapter is structured to gradually introduce you to new concepts, poses, and sequences. Begin at the start and move through the book at a pace that feels comfortable for you.

Utilize the Detailed Instructions: For each pose or sequence, there are detailed instructions aimed at ensuring your practice is both effective and safe. Pay close attention to these to get the most out of your practice.

Engage with the Bonus Material: The book includes bonus content designed to enrich your practice, including tips on nutrition, integrating mindfulness, and connecting with the chair yoga community.

Practice Regularly: Consistency is key to experiencing the full benefits of chair yoga. Aim to incorporate it into your daily routine, even if only for a few minutes a day.

Adapt as Needed: Listen to your body and feel free to adapt poses according to your comfort and ability. This book encourages making the practice your own.

Reflect on Your Journey: Use the book not only as a guide for your physical practice but also as a tool for reflection. Observe how your body and mind respond to chair yoga over time.

This book aims to be your companion on the journey toward improved physical and mental well-being through Chair Yoga. Whether you are new to yoga or adapting your existing practice, this guide seeks to empower you with knowledge, practice, and the confidence to explore the benefits of chair yoga for a healthier, more vibrant life.

Understanding Chair Yoga

What is Chair Yoga?

Chair Yoga is a form of yoga that modifies traditional yoga poses so they can be done while seated or using a chair for support. This adaptation makes yoga accessible to people who cannot stand for long periods, have limited mobility, or prefer a gentle approach to their practice. Chair Yoga encompasses a wide range of movements and exercises designed to stretch, flex, and strengthen the body, all while seated. It's an ideal way for seniors and individuals with physical limitations to enjoy the benefits of yoga, including improved flexibility, better posture, enhanced breathing, and stress reduction.

The Importance of Movement in Your 60s and Beyond

As we age, staying active becomes increasingly crucial for maintaining health and quality of life. Movement, especially in your 60s and beyond, is vital for several reasons:

- Maintaining Muscle Strength and Bone Density: Regular physical activity helps preserve muscle strength and bone density, reducing the risk of osteoporosis and falls.
- Enhancing Flexibility and Mobility: Keeping the body flexible and mobile is essential for performing everyday activities with ease and comfort.

- Improving Balance and Coordination: Exercise helps improve balance and coordination, crucial for preventing falls, a common concern among older adults.
- Supporting Cardiovascular Health: Physical activity supports heart health by improving circulation and reducing the risk of heart disease.
- Boosting Mental Health: Exercise has been shown to reduce symptoms of depression and anxiety, enhance cognitive function, and improve overall mood.
- Promoting Independence: Staying active is key to maintaining independence, allowing seniors to perform daily tasks and engage in their favorite activities.

Chair Yoga offers a safe, effective way to incorporate movement into your routine, regardless of your physical condition. By adapting yoga practices for the chair, it provides an accessible path to staying active, supporting not only physical health but also mental and emotional well-being. It's a testament to the idea that movement is beneficial at any age and that it's never too late to start improving your health through exercise.

Setting Up Your Space

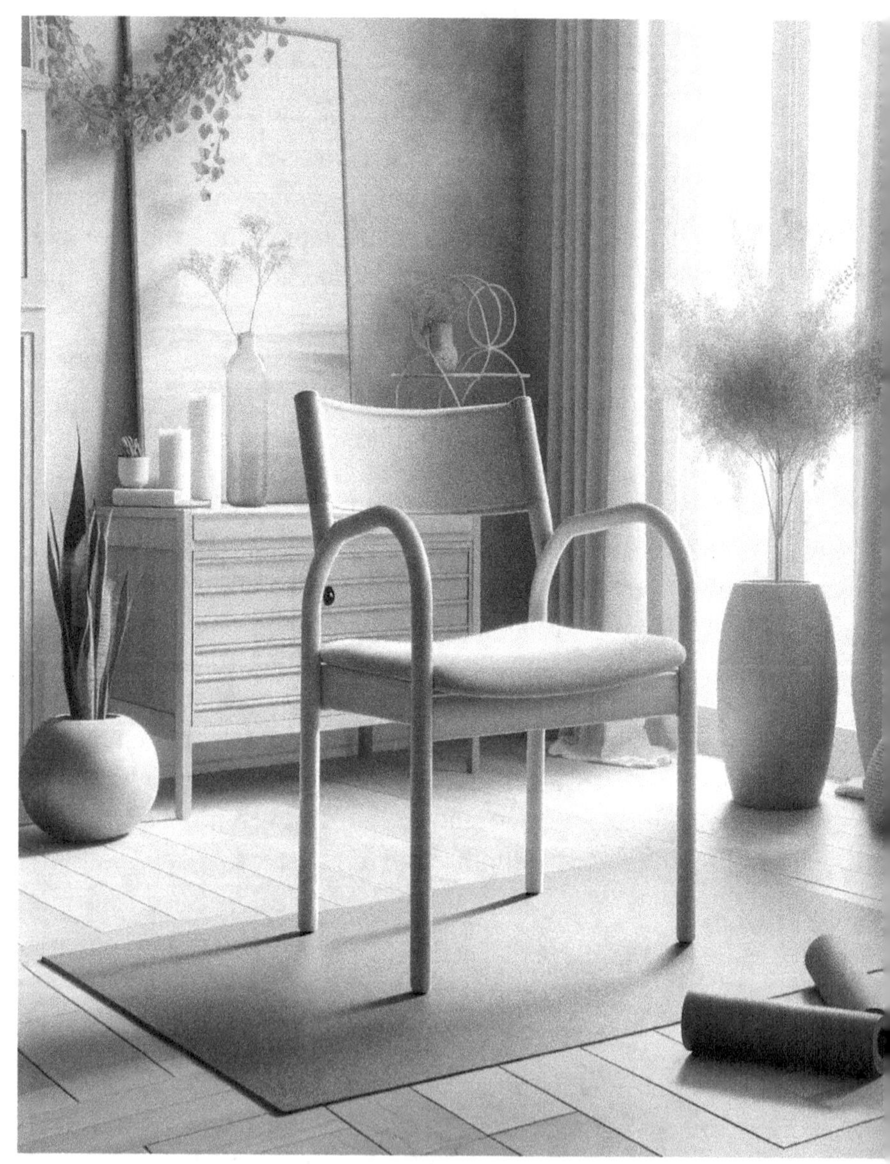

Creating a conducive environment for chair yoga enhances the experience, making each session more effective and enjoyable. Here are key considerations for setting up your space:

Choosing the Right Chair

Stability: Choose a sturdy chair that doesn't wobble, ensuring it can support your weight safely during different poses.

Armless Design: An armless chair is preferable as it allows for greater freedom of movement during exercises.

Proper Height: The chair should be at a height where your feet can rest flat on the ground when seated, with knees at a 90-degree angle. This alignment supports proper posture.

Creating a Safe and Inviting Yoga Space

Non-Slip Surface: Place your chair on a non-slip yoga mat or a stable, non-slippery floor to ensure the chair stays in place during your practice.

Adequate Space: Ensure there's enough room around your chair to move your arms freely and perform modified poses without constraints.

Minimal Distractions: Choose a quiet spot, away from high-traffic areas of your home, to maintain focus and relaxation.

Lighting and Ventilation: A well-lit and ventilated space contributes to a more pleasant and invigorating practice. Natural light and fresh air are especially beneficial.

Personal Touches: Adding elements like indoor plants, soft colors, or inspirational images can create a more peaceful and personalized environment.

Incorporating these elements into your chair yoga space can significantly enhance your practice, making it a sacred time for rejuvenation and self-care.

Safety First: Guidelines for Practicing Chair Yoga

Listening to Your Body

One of the most important aspects of practicing Chair Yoga, or any form of exercise, especially as you age, is to listen to your body. This means paying attention to the signals it sends you during your practice. If a pose or movement causes discomfort or pain, it's a sign to stop and adjust. Remember, yoga is not about pushing your limits to the point of pain but rather about enhancing your well-being through gentle stretching and strengthening.

Start Slowly: Especially if you're new to yoga or exercise in general, start with the most basic poses and gradually increase the intensity as your body adapts.

Recognize Your Limits: Acknowledge that some days you might be able to do more than on others. Respect your body's limitations on any given day.

Use the Breath as a Guide: Your breath can be a powerful indicator of how your body is coping with the poses. If you find your breath becoming short, strained, or uncomfortable, it may be time to ease up.

Modifying Poses for Comfort and Safety

Adaptation is key in Chair Yoga, allowing you to gain the benefits of each pose without risk of injury. Most yoga poses can be modified to fit your level of mobility and comfort.

Use Props: Props such as blocks, straps, or cushions can help adjust poses to your comfort level. For example, if reaching the floor is difficult, a block can bring the floor closer to you.

Adjust the Chair: Ensure the chair you use is stable and without wheels. Chairs with a flat seat and no arms are ideal, as they allow more freedom of movement.

Seek Guidance When Needed: If you're unsure how to modify a pose, seek advice from a qualified yoga instructor who has experience with chair yoga. They can offer personalized adjustments to suit your needs.

Creating a Safe Practice Environment

Ensure Stability: Practice on a non-slip surface to ensure your chair remains stable during your session. A yoga mat under the chair can provide additional grip.

Keep Space Clear: Ensure the area around your chair is clear of any objects or furniture you could bump into while moving.

Wear Appropriate Clothing: Wear comfortable clothing that allows for movement but is not so loose that it gets in the way or catches on the chair.

By adhering to these guidelines, you can enjoy a safe and beneficial Chair Yoga practice that supports your physical and mental health, fostering a sense of well-being and vitality.

Chapter Two: The Exercises

To ensure a comprehensive and accessible Chair Yoga practice, we'll cover a series of exercises designed to promote flexibility, strength, balance, and overall well-being. For each exercise, I'll provide a step-by-step guide along with an illustration to help you practice safely and effectively.

1. Seated Marching

Objective: Improves lower body strength and circulation.

Benefits:

- Enhances leg strength, focusing on the quadriceps and hamstrings.
- Boosts blood circulation in the lower extremities.
- Promotes coordination and balance while seated.

Steps:

1. Sit Up Straight: Begin by sitting on the edge of a stable chair without arms. Keep your back straight, shoulders relaxed, and feet flat on the ground, hip-width apart.

2. Engage Your Core: Gently engage your abdominal muscles by pulling your belly button towards your spine. This provides stability and support for your lower back.

3. Start Marching: Lift your right knee towards your chest as high as comfortably possible, then place it back on the ground. Repeat with your left knee. This movement mimics marching on the spot.

4. Maintain Posture: Keep your upper body stable and your back straight throughout the exercise. Avoid leaning backward or forward as you lift your knees.

5. Breathe: Inhale as you lift your knee, and exhale as you lower it back down. Maintaining a steady breath will help coordinate your movements andenhance the exercise's benefits.

6. Continue the Movement: Alternate between your right and left leg, gradually increasing your pace as you become more comfortable with the movement. Aim for 1-2 minutes of continuous seated marching, or as long as you can maintain good form.

Safety Tips:

- Ensure the chair is stable and will not slide or tip over.
- Start slow, especially if you're new to the exercise or have balance concerns.
- Stop the exercise if you feel any pain or discomfort.

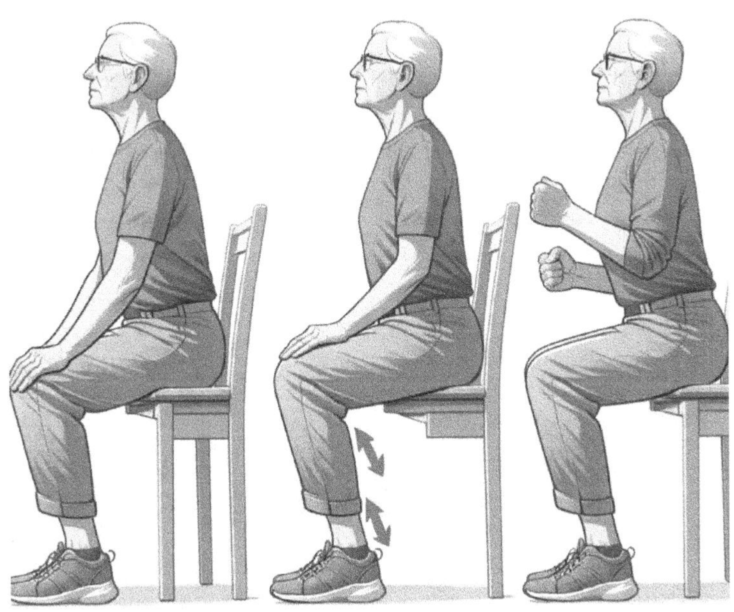

2. Chair Cat-Cow Stretch

Objective: Enhances spine flexibility and relieves tension in the back and neck.

Benefits:

- Increases flexibility in the spine and neck.
- Stimulates the abdominal organs, potentially aiding digestion.
- Relieves tension and stiffness in the back and neck.
- Encourages deep breathing, which enhances relaxation.

Steps:

1. Start in a Seated Neutral Position: Sit on the edge of a stable chair without arms, feet flat on the ground, and hands resting on your knees. Maintain a straight spine and relaxed shoulders.

2. Cow Pose (Inhalation): On an inhale, arch your back, pushing your chest forward and upward. Tilt your head back slightly, looking up toward the ceiling, allowing your belly to drop toward your thighs. This position encourages a gentle stretch across the front of your torso.

3. Cat Pose (Exhalation): On an exhale, round your spine, tucking your chin to your chest and pulling your belly in. Push your back toward the chair, creating a rounded spine like a cat stretching. This position helps to stretch the muscles in your back.

4. Flow Between Poses: Continue to alternate between the Cow Pose on your inhales and the Cat Pose on your exhales. Move smoothly and gently, allowing your breath to guide the movement.

5. Maintain Alignment: Keep your shoulders relaxed and away from your ears throughout the exercise. Focus on moving your spine vertebra by vertebra.

6. Repeat: Perform this flowing movement for 1-2 minutes, focusing on the sensation of flexibility and relief in your spine and back.

Safety Tips:

- Move gently and avoid overextending, especially if you have spine or neck issues.

- Keep movements fluid and aligned with your breath to prevent any jerky motions.

- If you experience any pain or discomfort, reduce the range of motion or stop the exercise.

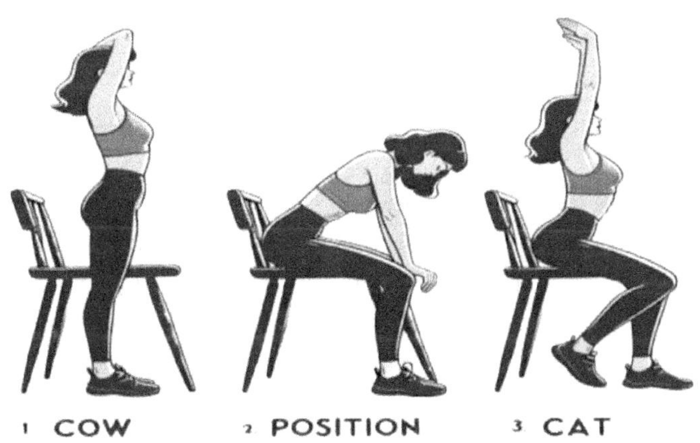

3. Seated Mountain Pose (Tadasana)

Objective: Builds posture and body awareness.

Benefits:

- ➤ Promotes a sense of groundedness and stability.
- ➤ Improves posture by aligning the spine and shoulders.
- ➤ Enhances focus and concentration.
- ➤ Serves as a foundation for other seated yoga poses.

Steps:

1. Find Your Seat: Sit on the edge of a stable chair without arms, feet planted firmly on the ground, hip-width apart. Ensure your knees are directly over your ankles.

2. Align Your Spine: Lengthen your spine as if a string is pulling you up from the top of your head. Draw your shoulders back and down, away from your ears, and face forward with your chin parallel to the floor.

3. Position Your Hands: Rest your hands on your thighs with palms down for grounding or turn them up to open up for receiving energy. Alternatively, you can join your hands in the prayer position at your heart center.

4. Engage Your Core: Gently engage your abdominal muscles by drawing your belly button towards your spine. This helps support your back and stabilizes your posture.

5. Breathe: Maintain this posture as you take several deep, slow breaths. Focus on the sensation of your feet pressing into the floor and your crown reaching towards the sky.

6. Hold and Release: Hold the pose for 30 seconds to 1 minute, breathing deeply. To release, relax your hands and sit back comfortably in your chair.

Safety Tips:

+ Keep your feet firmly grounded to avoid straining your legs.
+ If you have lower back issues, be cautious not to overarch your spine.
+ Adjust the pose as needed to avoid any discomfort.

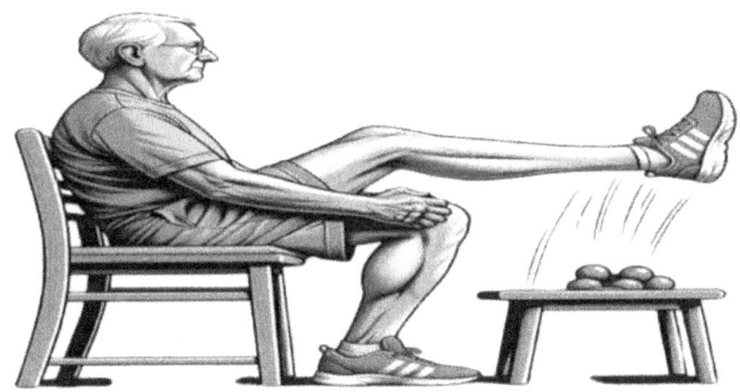

4. Seated Forward Bend (Paschimottanasana)

Objective: Stretches the spine and shoulders, promoting flexibility and relieving tension.

Benefits:

- Enhances spinal flexibility and stretches the back muscles.
- Relieves tension in the spine, neck, and shoulders.
- Stimulates the abdominal organs.
- Calms the mind and reduces stress.

Steps:

1. Begin in Seated Mountain Pose: Sit on the edge of a stable chair without arms, feet flat on the floor, and spine elongated.

2. Inhale and Extend: Inhale deeply, extending your arms overhead, stretching your spine upward.

3. Exhale and Bend Forward: Exhale as you hinge forward from your hips, keeping your back straight. Extend your hands toward your feet or place them on your shins or knees, depending on your flexibility.

4. Relax Your Neck: Allow your head to hang gently, relaxing your neck. Your gaze should be down towards your legs.

5. Hold the Pose: Stay in this forward bend, breathing deeply for 5-10 breaths. With each exhale, allow yourself to deepen into the stretch gently.

6. Return to Seated: Inhale as you slowly lift your torso back to the seated mountain pose, arms reaching overhead, and then exhale your arms down.

Safety Tips:

- Move into and out of the pose slowly to avoid dizziness.
- Keep the spine long throughout the bend to avoid compressing the vertebrae.
- If you have lower back issues, proceed cautiously, and consider using a supportive prop like a cushion or yoga block.

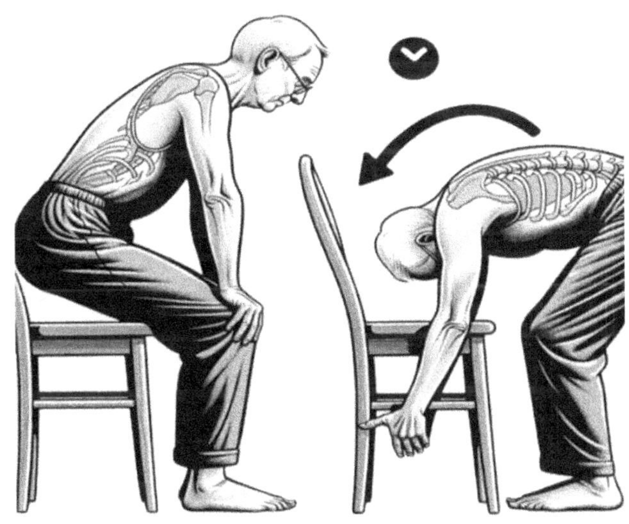

5. Chair Pigeon Pose

Objective: Opens up the hips and stretches the thighs, promoting flexibility and relieving tension in the lower body.

Benefits:

- ✓ Improves hip flexibility and mobility.
- ✓ Reduces tightness in the lower back and hips.
- ✓ Aids in alleviating symptoms of sciatica.
- ✓ Encourages a gentle stretch in the thighs and glutes.

Steps:

1. Start in Seated Mountain Pose: Sit on the edge of a stable chair without arms, with your feet flat on the floor and spine tall.

2. Prepare for Pigeon Pose: Lift your right ankle and place it on your left thigh, just above the knee. Keep your right knee in line with your right ankle as much as possible.

3. Adjust Your Posture: Ensure your spine is straight and tall. Gently press down on your right thigh with your right hand to deepen the stretch, if comfortable. Avoid pushing too hard to prevent strain.

4. Hold and Breathe: Stay in this position, breathing deeply for 5-10 breaths. Focus on relaxing your hip and thigh muscles with each exhale.

5. Switch Sides: Gently lower your right foot back to the floor and repeat the pose with your left ankle on your right thigh.

6. Return to Starting Position: After completing both sides, return to the Seated Mountain Pose and relax.

- Keep your foot flexed to protect your knee.
- If you feel any sharp pain, especially in the knee or hip, gently exit the pose.
- Use your hand for gentle pressure only; the aim is a stretch, not force.

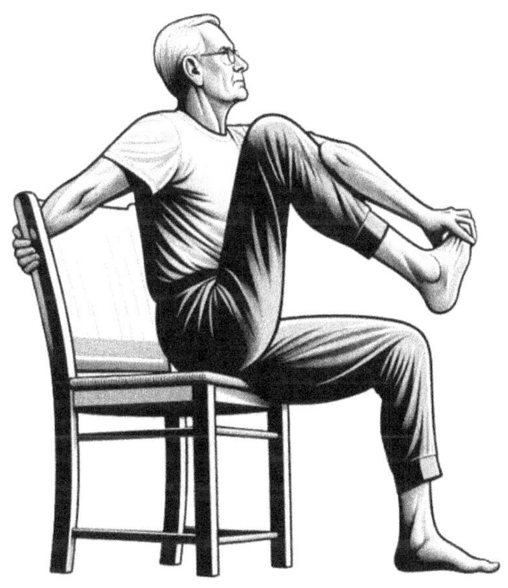

6. Seated Spinal Twist

Objective: Increases spinal mobility and can aid in digestion.

Benefits:

- ✓ Enhances spinal flexibility and stretches the back muscles.
- ✓ Stimulates the abdominal organs, potentially aiding digestion.
- ✓ Relieves tension in the spine, shoulders, and neck.
- ✓ Promotes detoxification and stimulates circulation.

Steps:

1. Start in Seated Mountain Pose: Sit on the edge of a stable chair without arms, with your feet flat on the floor and spine elongated.

2. Initiate the Twist: Turn your torso to the right, placing your left hand on the outside of your right knee and your right hand on the back of the chair or the seat beside you, depending on what feels comfortable and allows for a deeper twist.

3. Deepen the Twist: Inhale to lengthen your spine further, and as you exhale, gently deepen into the twist. Aim to keep your hips facing forward to ensure the twist originates from your mid and upper spine.

4. Maintain and Breathe: Hold this position, breathing deeply for 5-10 breaths. With each exhale, see if you can twist a little deeper, keeping the movement gentle and controlled.

5. Return to Center: Inhale as you slowly come back to facing forward, returning to your starting position.

6. Repeat on the Opposite Side: Turn your torso to the left, repeating the steps to twist in the opposite direction.

Safety Tips:

- Move into and out of the twist slowly to maintain balance and prevent strain.
- Keep the twist gentle; the goal is to feel a comfortable stretch, not to push to the point of discomfort.
- If you have any spinal injuries or conditions, proceed with caution and consult a healthcare professional if necessary.

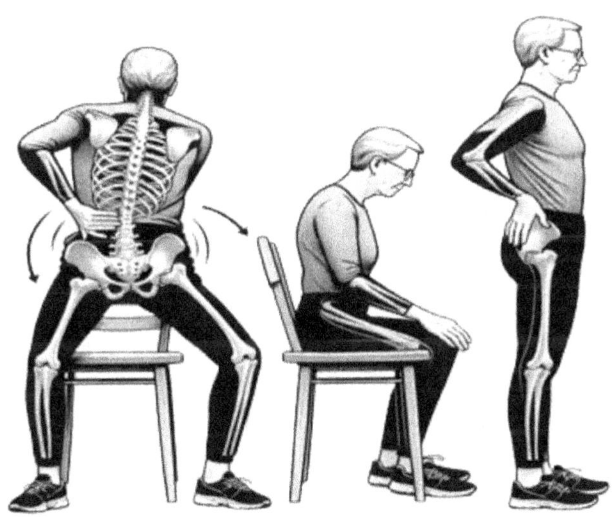

7. Seated Side Stretch

Objective: Stretches the side body and improves flexibility.

Benefits:

- ✓ Lengthens the muscles along the side of the torso, enhancing flexibility.
- ✓ Improves posture by opening up the ribcage and shoulders.
- ✓ Aids in breathing capacity by stretching the intercostal muscles.
- ✓ Relieves tension in the shoulders and neck.

Steps:

1. Begin in Seated Mountain Pose: Sit on the edge of a stable chair without arms, feet flat on the ground, and spine tall.

2. Initiate the Stretch: Place your right hand on the right side of the chair seat or hold onto the chair for support.

3. Extend and Stretch: Inhale and extend your left arm straight up by your ear. On the exhale, lean your torso to the right, keeping your left arm over your head, creating a deep stretch along the left side of your body.

4. Maintain Alignment: Keep your hips anchored to the chair and avoid leaning forward or backward. The stretch should come from the side of your torso.

5. Hold and Breathe: Hold the stretch for 5-10 breaths, focusing on deepening the stretch with each exhale.

6. Keep your neck in a neutral position, or gently turn your gaze up towards the ceiling to intensify the stretch.

7. Return to Center: Inhale and gently come back to an upright position, lowering your left arm.

8. Repeat on the Other Side: Repeat the stretch on the opposite side by placing your left hand on the chair, extending your right arm, and leaning to the left.

Safety Tips:

+ Move into and out of the stretch gently to avoid any sudden movements.
+ Keep the stretch comfortable; do not overextend to the point of discomfort.
+ Be mindful of your balance and ensure the chair is stable throughout the exercise.

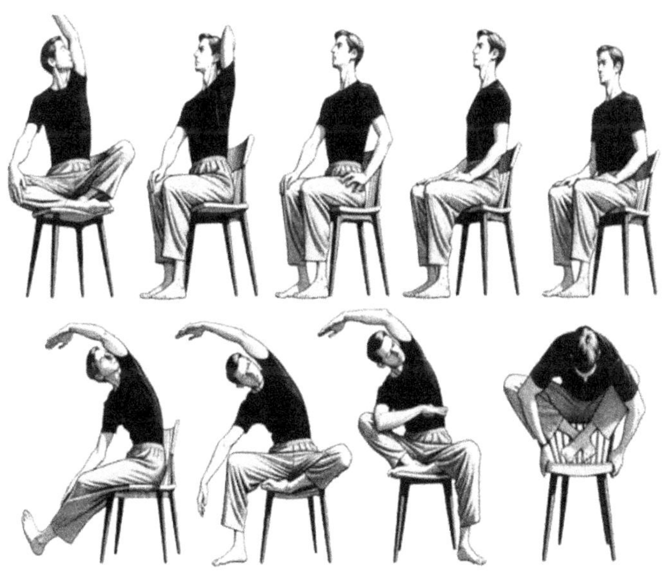

8. Wrist and Finger Stretches

Objective: Reduces the risk of carpal tunnel and keeps joints flexible.

Benefits:

- ✓ Improves flexibility and range of motion in the wrists and fingers.
- ✓ Relieves tension and stiffness in the hands, wrists, and forearms.
- ✓ Helps prevent conditions like carpal tunnel syndrome and arthritis-related discomfort.
- ✓ Enhances strength and dexterity in the hands and fingers.

Steps:

1. Begin in Seated Mountain Pose: Sit comfortably on the chair with your feet flat on the ground and your spine tall.

2. Extend Your Arms: Stretch both arms forward at shoulder height, palms facing down.

3. Wrist Flexion and Extension:

   Flexion: Gently bend your wrists down, pointing your fingers towards the floor. Hold for a few breaths, then release.

   Extension: Bend your wrists up, pointing your fingers towards the ceiling. Hold for a few breaths, then release.

4. Finger Stretches: Extend your fingers wide, stretching them apart, then make a fist. Repeat several times to enhance flexibility and circulation.

5. Wrist Circles: With your arms extended, rotate your wrists in circular motions, first in one direction, then the opposite. This helps to loosen up the joint.

6. Palm Stretch: With one hand, gently press back on the fingers of the opposite hand to stretch the palm and wrist. Switch hands and repeat.

Safety Tips:

- Perform the stretches gently to avoid overextending the joints.
- If you experience any pain or discomfort, reduce the intensity or discontinue the stretch
- Keep your movements slow and controlled, focusing on the sensation of stretching.

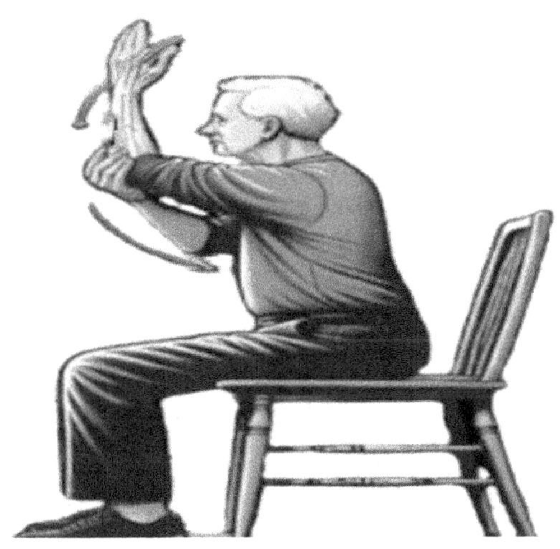

9. Ankle Circles

Objective: Improves ankle flexibility and circulation.

Benefits:

- ✓ Enhances range of motion and flexibility in the ankles.
- ✓ Promotes better circulation in the lower legs, which is beneficial for reducing swelling and preventing venous issues.
- ✓ Strengthens the muscles around the ankles, supporting overall balance and mobility.
- ✓ Relieves tension and stiffness in the ankle joints.

Steps:

1. Sit Comfortably: Begin in a seated position on a chair, with your back straight and feet flat on the floor.

2. Extend One Leg: Lift your right leg and extend it out in front of you, keeping the leg as straight as possible. Rest your heel on the edge of the floor or on a low stool, with your toes pointing upwards.

3. Rotate Your Ankle: Slowly rotate your right ankle in a circular motion, first clockwise for 5-10 rotations, then counter-clockwise for 5-10 rotations. Focus on making smooth, controlled circles.

4. Switch Legs: Lower your right leg back to the starting position. Repeat the ankle circles with your left leg, ensuring equal time and rotations for both ankles.

5. Flex and Point: For an added stretch, flex your foot
    to point your toes upwards, then point your toes
    away from you. Repeat this movement several times
    to stretch the calves and shins.

Safety Tips:

- Keep your movements gentle and controlled to
  avoid straining the muscles around your ankles.
- If you experience any pain or discomfort, reduce the
  range of motion or stop the exercise.
- Ensure you perform the exercise on both ankles to
  maintain balance and symmetry in flexibility and
  strength.

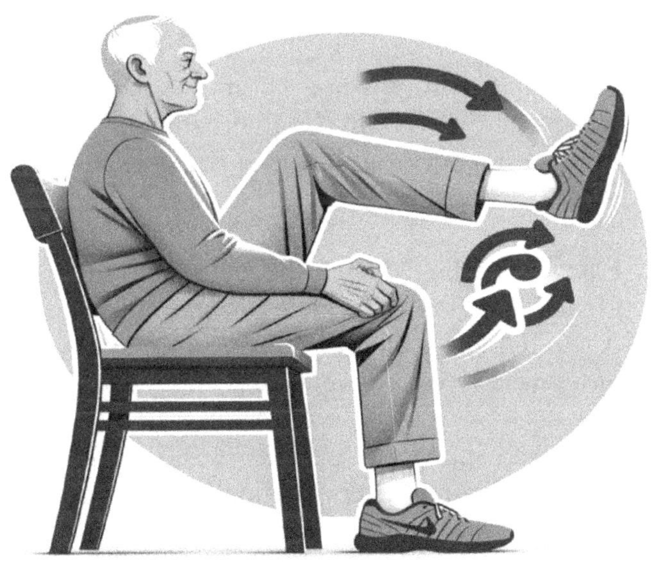

10. Leg Extensions

Objective: Strengthens the quadriceps and improves knee mobility.

Benefits:

- ✓ Builds strength in the quadriceps, which are key for walking, standing, and maintaining balance.
- ✓ Enhances the flexibility and range of motion of the knee joints.
- ✓ Can help alleviate stiffness and improve circulation in the lower legs.
- ✓ Supports overall leg health and functionality.

Steps

1. Start in a Seated Position: Sit on the edge of a chair with your feet flat on the floor, spine straight, and hands resting on your thighs or the sides of the chair for balance.

2. Extend One Leg: Slowly lift your right foot off the ground, straightening the leg in front of you until it is parallel to the floor. Flex your foot to point your toes towards you, engaging the muscles in your leg.

3. Hold and Lower: Hold the position for a few seconds, feeling the contraction in your quadriceps. Slowly lower your leg back to the starting position.

4. Repeat: Perform 10-15 repetitions with your right leg before switching to your left leg. Aim for 2-3 sets on each leg.

5. Breathing: Maintain steady breathing throughout the exercise. Inhale as you prepare to lift your leg, and exhale as you extend it. Inhale again as you return to the starting position.

+ Ensure the chair is stable and will not slip or move during the exercise.
+ If you experience any pain, especially in the knees, reduce the range of motion or discontinue the exercise.
+ Keep the movements controlled and slow to maximize muscle engagement and prevent injury.

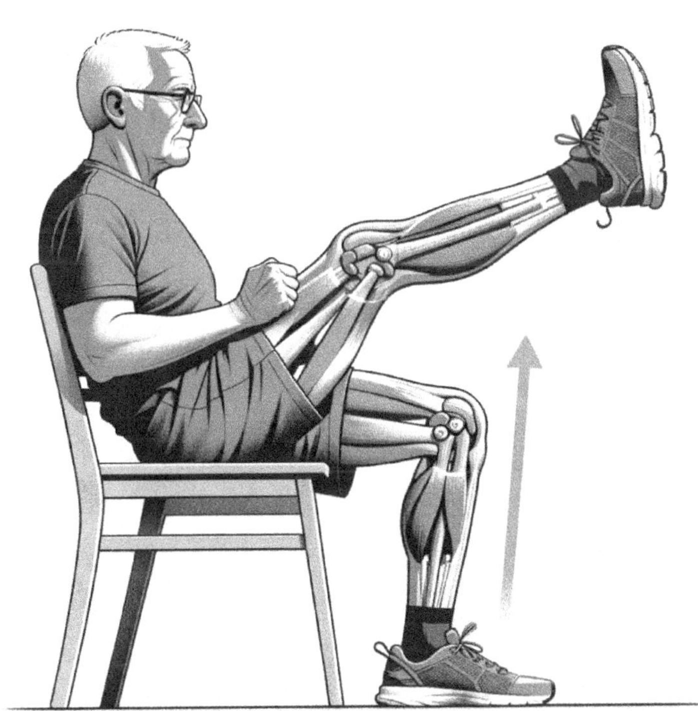

11. Arm Circles

Objective: Warms up and strengthens the shoulders.

Benefits:

- ✓ Increases mobility and flexibility in the shoulders.
- ✓ Warms up the upper body for further exercise, reducing the risk of injury.
- ✓ Enhances muscular endurance and strength in the shoulder area.
- ✓ Promotes blood circulation in the arms and shoulders.

Steps:

1. Start Seated: Sit on a chair with your feet flat on the ground, and spine straight.

2. Extend Your Arms: Extend your arms straight out to the sides at shoulder height, palms facing down.

3. Perform Small Circles: Begin by rotating your arms in small circles forward for 30 seconds.

4. Switch Directions: After 30 seconds, reverse the direction and rotate your arms in small circles backward for another 30 seconds.

5. Increase the Size: Gradually increase the diameter of the circles until you're making as large circles as comfortable, continuing for 30 seconds in each direction.

6. Relax: Lower your arms and relax for a few moments before repeating, if desired.

- Keep your movements controlled and avoid jerky motions to prevent shoulder strain.
- Start with smaller circles, gradually increasing the size as your shoulders warm up.
- If you experience any pain, stop the exercise and rest.

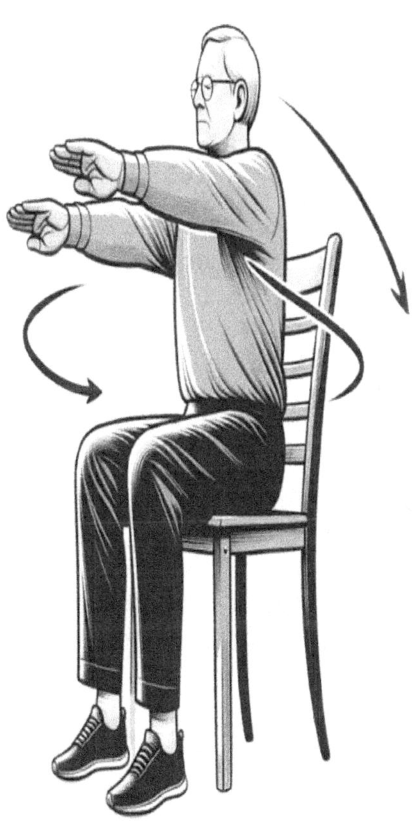

12. Shoulder Shrugs

Objective: Releases tension in the shoulders and neck.

Benefits:

- ✓ Relieves tension and stiffness in the shoulder and neck area.
- ✓ Improves range of motion and flexibility in the shoulders.
- ✓ Can help reduce headaches and upper body discomfort related to stress.
- ✓ Strengthens the muscles around the shoulders.

Steps:

1. Sit Comfortably: Sit on a chair with your feet flat on the floor and your spine straight. Relax your arms by your sides or place them on your lap.

2. Shrug Your Shoulders: Inhale and lift your shoulders towards your ears as high as you comfortably can, engaging the trapezius muscles.

3. Hold and Release: Hold the shrug for a moment, then exhale and release your shoulders down, feeling the tension melting away.

4. Repeat: Perform 10-15 shoulder shrugs, focusing on the sensation of tension release with each downward movement.

5. Maintain Good Posture: Keep your spine straight and your neck in a neutral position throughout the exercise to maximize benefits.

- Perform the shrugs with controlled motion to avoid strain.
- If you experience any discomfort or pain, reduce the range of motion or stop the exercise.
- Breathe naturally and avoid holding your breath.

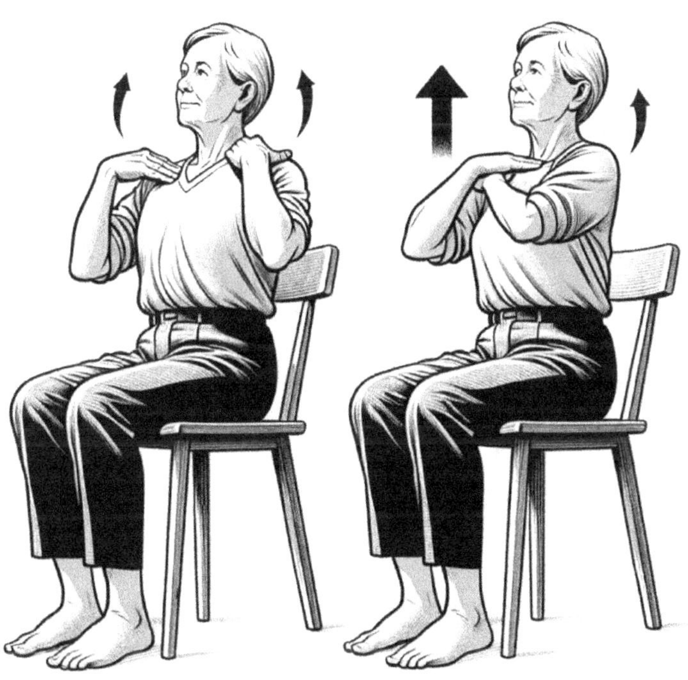

13. Neck Stretch

Objective: Relieves neck tension and improves flexibility.

Benefits:

- ✓ Eases tension and stiffness in the neck muscles.
- ✓ Increases flexibility and range of motion in the neck.
- ✓ Can help alleviate headaches and neck pain associated with poor posture.
- ✓ Promotes relaxation and stress relief.

Steps:

1. Begin in a Seated Position: Sit comfortably on a chair with your feet flat on the floor and your spine straight. Relax your shoulders down away from your ears.

2. Side Neck Stretch:
   - Gently tilt your head to the right, bringing your right ear towards your right shoulder. Keep your left shoulder relaxed and avoid lifting it towards your ear.
   - Place your right hand gently on your head to add a slight amount of pressure, increasing the stretch on the left side of your neck. Keep the left arm relaxed by your side or on your lap.
   - Hold for 15-30 seconds, breathing deeply and focusing on the stretch.
   - Slowly release and return to the starting position. Repeat on the left side.

3. Forward Neck Stretch:

- Gently lower your chin towards your chest, feeling a stretch along the back of your neck.

- Place both hands on the back of your head to add a slight amount of pressure, deepening the stretch.
- Hold for 15-30 seconds, breathing deeply.
- Slowly release and lift your head back to the starting position.

- Perform the stretches gently and avoid overstretching to prevent strain.
- Keep your movements slow and controlled, especially when applying pressure with your hands.
- If you experience any pain or discomfort, reduce the intensity of the stretch or stop the exercise.

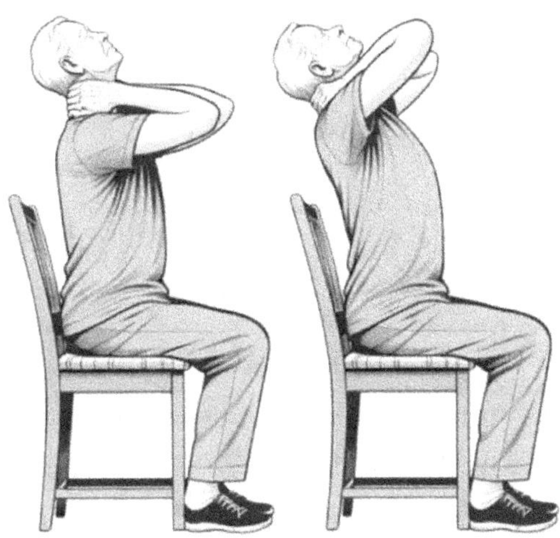

14. Upper Body Twist

Objective: Engages and strengthens the core and waist.

Benefits:
- ✓ Improves spinal mobility and flexibility.
- ✓ Strengthens core muscles, including the obliques and lower back.
- ✓ Helps in digestion and stimulates abdominal organs.
- ✓ Reduces tension in the back and improves posture.

Steps:
1. Start Seated: Sit on the edge of the chair with your feet flat on the floor, hip-width apart. Keep your spine straight and tall.

2. Initiate the Twist: Place your right hand on the back of the chair. Bring your left hand to your right knee or the outside of your right thigh.

3. Twist Your Upper Body: As you inhale, lengthen your spine further. On the exhale, gently twist your torso to the right, keeping your hips facing forward. The twist should come from the waist up.

4. Hold and Deepen: Hold the twist for 15-30 seconds, deepening the stretch with each exhale. Keep your shoulders down and relaxed.

5. Return to Center: Inhale as you slowly return to the starting position.

6. Repeat on the Other Side: Repeat the twist on the left side, with your left hand behind you and your right hand on your left knee or thigh.

Safety Tips
- Ensure your movements are slow and controlled to prevent any strain.
- Keep the twist gentle; do not force it beyond your comfortable range of motion.
- If you have any spine or back issues, proceed with caution and consult a healthcare provider if necessary.

15. Toe Taps

Objective: Strengthens leg muscles and improves lower body circulation.

Benefits:
- ✓ Enhances circulation in the lower extremities, which can help reduce swelling and prevent venous issues.
- ✓ Strengthens the muscles in the lower legs, including the calves and shins.
- ✓ Improves coordination and mobility in the feet and ankles.
- ✓ Can aid in maintaining balance and preventing falls by strengthening the lower body.

Steps:
1. Start Seated: Sit on the edge of a chair with your feet flat on the ground, hip-width apart. Keep your back straight and your hands on your thighs or the sides of the chair for balance.

2. Perform Toe Taps: Lift the toes of your right foot as high as you can, keeping your heel on the ground. Then, lower your toes and lift your heel, tapping the toes on the ground. Continue this toe-heel tapping motion.

3. 3.Maintain Control: Focus on controlled movements, engaging the muscles in your lower legs. Keep the rest of your body still and stable.

4. Switch Feet: After completing a set of 10-15
   taps with your right foot, switch to your left
   foot and repeat the exercise.

5. Repeat: Aim for 2-3 sets per foot, depending
   on your comfort and fitness level.

Safety Tips:
- Ensure your chair is stable and will not move
  during the exercise.
- If you feel any pain or discomfort, especially
  in the ankles or feet, stop the exercise.
- Keep your movements slow and controlled to
  maximize muscle engagement and prevent
  strain.

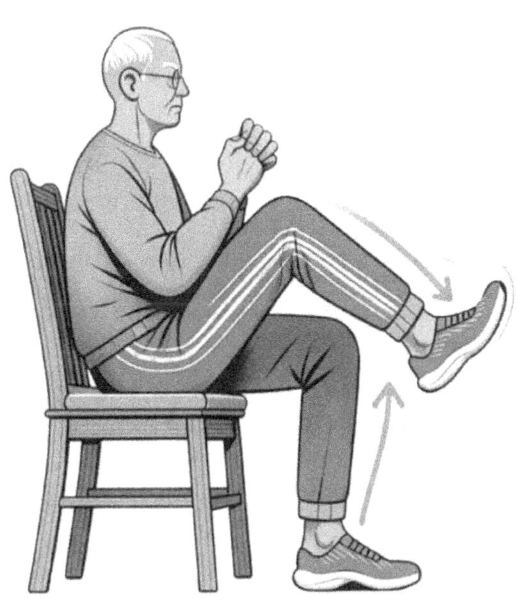

16. Heel Raises

Objective: Strengthens calves and improves ankle stability.
Benefits:

- ✓ Enhances strength in the calf muscles, which support walking, running, and standing.
- ✓ Improves stability and balance by strengthening the ankles.
- ✓ Can help prevent ankle injuries by improving flexibility and resilience.
- ✓ Promotes circulation in the lower legs, reducing the risk of swelling and venous issues.

Steps:

1. Start in a Seated Position: Sit on the edge of a chair with your feet flat on the ground, hip-width apart. Keep your back straight and your hands on your thighs or the sides of the chair for balance.

2. Perform the Heel Raises: Press down through the balls of your feet to lift your heels off the ground as high as you comfortably can, engaging your calf muscles.

3. Hold and Lower: Hold the raised position for a moment, then slowly lower your heels back to the ground.

4. Repeat: Perform 10-15 heel raises, focusing on controlled, smooth movements. Aim for 2-3 sets, depending on your comfort and fitness level.

5.

- Ensure the chair is stable and will not slip during the exercise.
- If you experience any pain or discomfort, especially in the calves or ankles, stop the exercise.
- Keep the movements controlled to maximize muscle engagement and prevent strain.

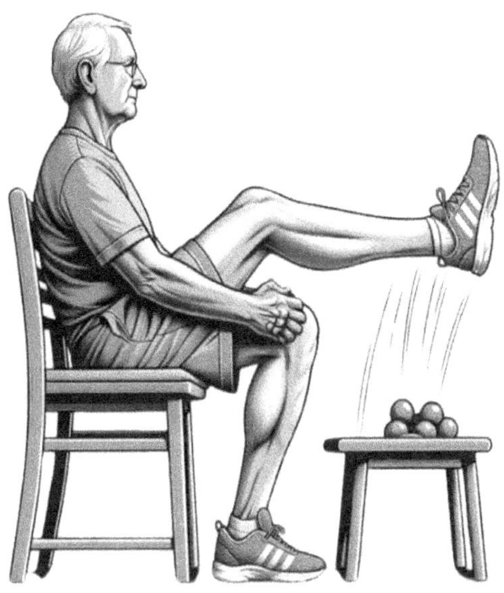

17. Seated Leg Lifts

Objective: Strengthens the abs and legs.

Benefits:

- ✓ Engages and strengthens the core muscles, including the lower abdominals.
- ✓ Improves leg strength and stability.
- ✓ Enhances coordination and balance.
- ✓ Promotes lower body circulation.

Steps:

1. Start in a Seated Position: Sit on the edge of a chair with your back straight, feet flat on the ground, and hands holding the sides of the chair for support.

2. Lift One Leg: Slowly lift your right leg, keeping it as straight as possible, to a height that feels comfortable but challenging. Aim to lift so your leg is parallel to the ground or as close as possible.

3. Engage Your Core: As you lift your leg, focus on engaging your abdominal muscles to maintain balance and stability. Keep your back straight and avoid leaning backward.

4. Hold and Lower: Hold your leg in the lifted position for a few seconds, then slowly lower it back to the starting position.

5. Repeat with the Other Leg: Perform the same movement with your left leg.

6. Do Several Repetitions: Aim for 10-15 repetitions per leg, depending on your fitness level. Consider performing 2-3 sets for a more challenging workout.

- Ensure the chair is stable and will not slide or tip over during the exercise.
- Move slowly and with control to prevent jerky movements that could strain muscles.
- If you experience any pain, especially in the lower back or knees, reduce the height of the leg lift or stop the exercise.

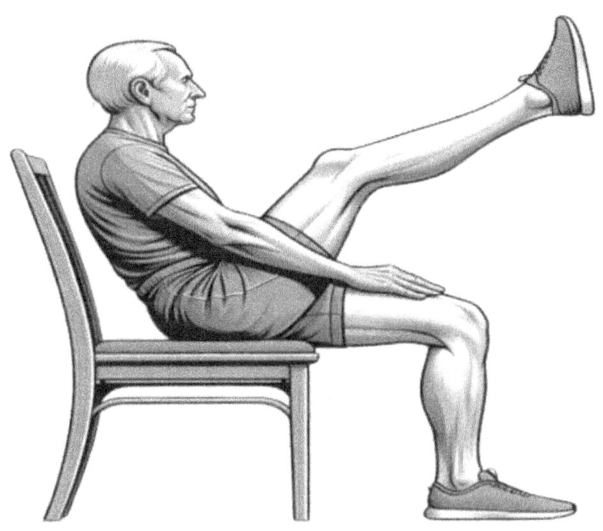

18. Seated Knee Lifts with a Twist

Objective: Engages the core and obliques.
Benefits:

- ✓ Strengthens the abdominal muscles, focusing on the obliques.
- ✓ Enhances spinal rotation mobility.
- ✓ Improves balance and coordination.
- ✓ Stimulates digestion and abdominal organs.

1. **Steps:**
   1. Start in a Seated Position: Sit on the edge of a chair with your feet flat on the ground, hip-width apart. Keep your back straight and your hands behind your head with elbows wide.

   2. Lift and Twist: Lift your right knee towards your chest while simultaneously twisting your torso so your left elbow moves towards the lifted knee. Aim to engage your obliques as you twist.

   3. Return to Center: Slowly lower your right leg back to the starting position while unwinding your torso to face forward again.

   4. Alternate Sides: Repeat the movement with your left knee and twist towards it with your right elbow.

5. Continue Alternating: Perform 10-15 repetitions on each side, alternating smoothly and focusing on the twist and lift with each repetition.

6. Keep Engaged: Ensure your core is engaged throughout the exercise to maximize benefits and support your spine.

Safety Tips:

- Move slowly and with control to avoid any jerky movements that could strain your back or neck.
- Keep your movements within a comfortable range of motion to avoid overstretching.
- If you experience any discomfort or pain, particularly in the back or neck, stop the exercise.

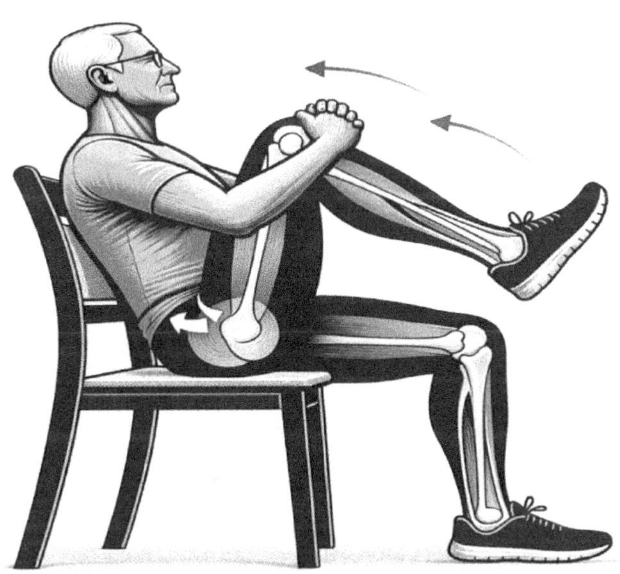

19. Chair Supported Squat

Objective: Builds leg and glute strength.

Benefits:

- ✓ Strengthens the quadriceps, hamstrings, and glutes.
- ✓ Enhances balance and stability by engaging core muscles.
- ✓ Improves flexibility in the hips and knees.
- ✓ Can aid in performing daily activities more easily, like sitting down and standing up.

Steps:

1.Start Standing: Stand in front of a chair with your feet hip-width apart, toes slightly turned out. Ensure the chair is stable and won't move.

2. Initiate the Squat: Extend your arms in front of you for balance. Begin to lower your body by bending your knees, pushing your hips back as if you're going to sit down on the chair.

3. Touchdown Lightly: Gently touch the chair with your buttocks but do not fully sit. Keep your weight in your heels and your core engaged.

4. Rise Up: Press through your heels to return to the standing position, squeezing your glutes as you rise.

5. Repeat: Perform 10-15 squats, focusing on form and control. Aim for 2-3 sets.

Safety Tips:

- Keep your chest lifted and back straight throughout the squat to avoid straining your lower back.
- Ensure your knees do not extend beyond your toes to prevent knee strain.
- If you have balance issues, keep the chair close for support.

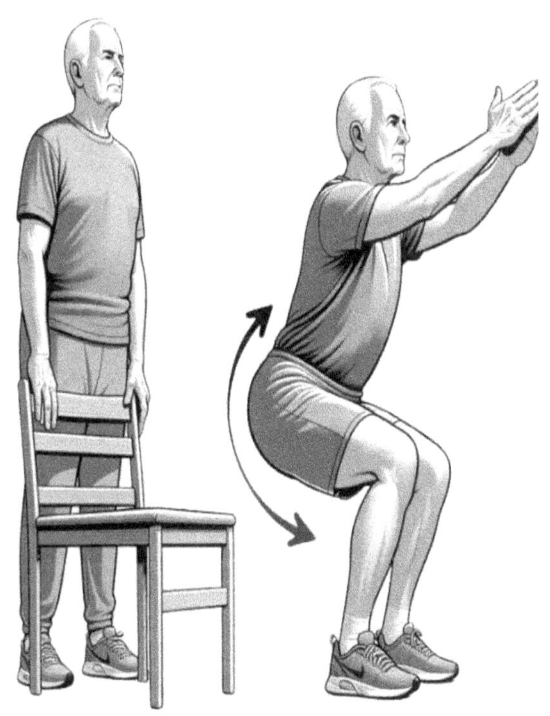

20. Seated "T" Pose

Objective: Strengthens the upper back and shoulders.

Benefits:

- ✓ Enhances shoulder stability and mobility.
- ✓ Strengthens the muscles of the upper back, contributing to better posture.
- ✓ Reduces the risk of shoulder and back pain by promoting muscular balance.
- ✓ Can improve the range of motion and flexibility in the shoulders.

Steps:

1. Start in a Seated Position: Sit on the edge of a chair with your feet flat on the ground, hip-width apart. Keep your spine straight and tall.

2. Extend Your Arms: Extend your arms to the sides at shoulder height, palms facing down, to form a "T" with your body.

3. Engage Your Back: Focus on squeezing your shoulder blades together as if you're trying to hold a pencil between them. This engages the muscles in your upper back.

4. Hold the Pose: Hold this position, keeping your arms strong and straight, for 15-30 seconds. Keep your neck long and your gaze forward.

5. Release: Gently lower your arms back to your sides and relax your shoulders.

6. Repeat: Perform 2-3 sets, resting briefly between each set to prevent fatigue.

- Keep your movements controlled and avoid lifting your arms beyond shoulder height to prevent strain.
- If you experience any pain or discomfort in your shoulders or back, lower your arms and rest.
- Breathe evenly throughout the exercise to maintain relaxation and focus.

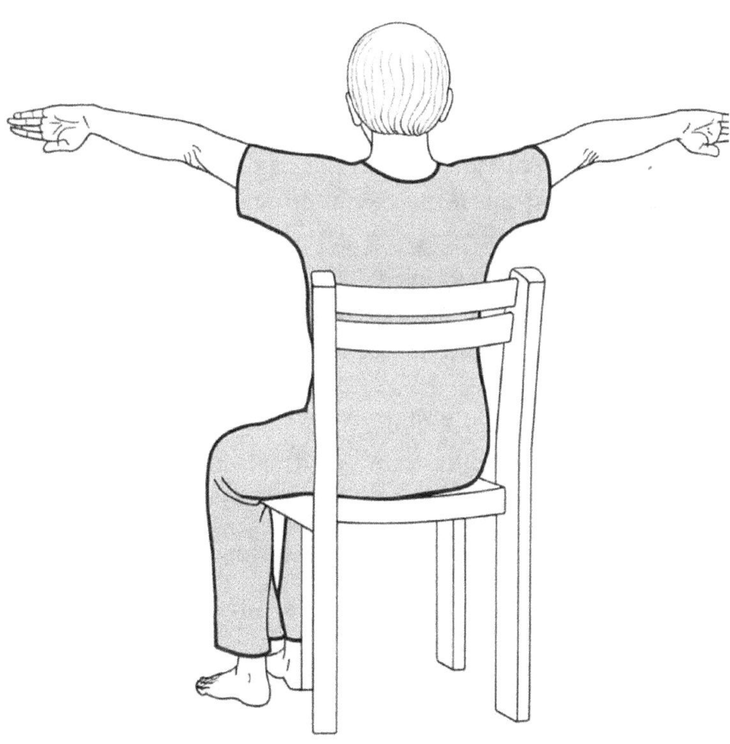

21. Seated Bicycle Crunches

Objective: To engage and strengthen the core muscles, with a focus on the obliques and rectus abdominis, from a seated position.

Benefits:

- ✓ Enhances core stability and strength.
- ✓ Promotes better posture and spinal alignment.
- ✓ Stimulates the abdominal organs, aiding in digestion.

Steps:

1. Position Yourself: Sit on the edge of a chair with your feet flat on the floor. Lean slightly back, holding onto the sides of the chair for support.

2. Lift Your Legs: Lift your feet off the floor, bringing your knees towards your chest.

3. Perform the Crunches: Extend your left leg out in front of you while simultaneously twisting your torso to bring your right elbow towards your left knee. Then switch sides, extending your right leg while twisting to bring your left elbow towards your right knee. Continue alternating sides in a pedaling motion.

4. Breathe: Inhale as you extend the leg and exhale during the twist to engage the core muscles fully.

5. Repetitions: Aim for 10-15 repetitions on each side, or as many as you can do with good form.

- Ensure the chair is stable and won't move during the exercise.
- Keep movements controlled to avoid strain on the lower back.
- If you experience any discomfort, reduce the range of motion or take a break.

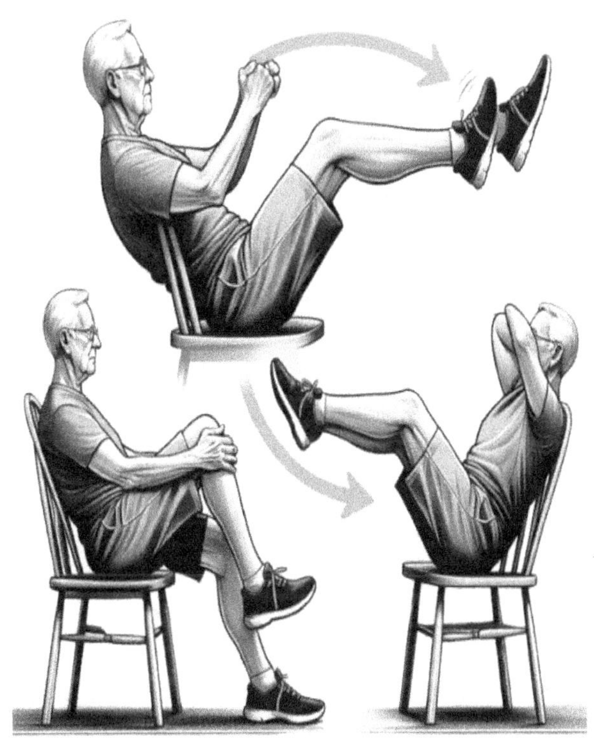

22. Arm and Leg Lifts

Objective: Enhances coordination and balance while simultaneously strengthening the limbs.

Benefits:

- ✓ Improves limb strength and stability.
- ✓ Enhances coordination between different parts of the body.
- ✓ Promotes balance, which is crucial for preventing falls.
- ✓ Engages both the upper and lower body in a single exercise.

Steps:

1. Sit Securely: Sit on the edge of a stable chair with your feet flat on the floor and your spine in a neutral position.

2. Lift Arm and Opposite Leg: Lift your right arm overhead while simultaneously lifting your left leg straight out in front of you. Try to keep both your arm and leg as straight as possible.

3. Hold the Position: Hold this position for a few seconds, focusing on balancing and stabilizing your body.

4. Return to Starting Position: Gently lower your arm and leg back to the starting position.

5. Switch Sides: Repeat the movement with your left arm and right leg.

6. Perform Repetitions: Aim for 10-15 repetitions on each side, or as many as comfortable, focusing on smooth, controlled movements.

- Ensure the chair is stable and won't slide or tip over during the exercise.
- Start with slow movements to maintain balance and prevent any strain.
- If lifting both an arm and leg simultaneously is too challenging, start by lifting one limb at a time and gradually progress as you become more comfortable.

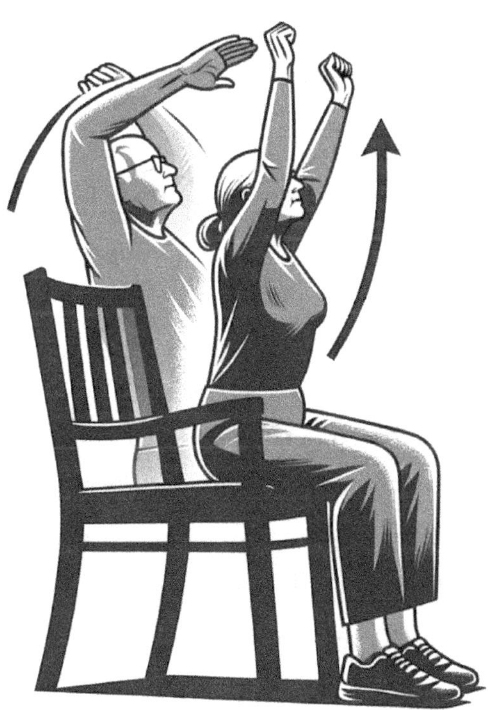

23. Wrist Flexor and Extensor Stretches

Objective: To increase flexibility and range of motion in the wrists and forearms.

Benefits:

- ✓ Reduces stiffness and risk of injuries in the wrist and forearm area.
- ✓ Improves grip strength and the ability to perform daily tasks with ease.
- ✓ Aids in the prevention of conditions like carpal tunnel syndrome and tendonitis.

Steps for Wrist Flexor Stretch:

1. Start Seated: Sit comfortably on a chair with your feet flat on the floor and your spine straight.

2. Extend Your Arm: Extend one arm forward at shoulder height, palm facing up.

3. Apply Gentle Pressure: Use the other hand to gently press down on the fingers of the extended arm, feeling a stretch in the underside of your forearm.

4. Hold the Stretch: Hold this position for 15-30 seconds, taking deep breaths.

5. Switch Arms: Repeat the stretch with the other arm.

Steps for Wrist Extensor Stretch:

1. Extend Your Arm: With your arm extended forward and palm facing down, use the other hand to gently press the fingers towards the floor.

2. Hold the Stretch: Maintain the position for 15-30 seconds, focusing on the stretch along the top of your forearm.

3. Switch Arms: Perform the stretch on the opposite arm.

Safety Tips:

- Perform the stretches gently to avoid overextending the muscles.
- If you experience any sharp pain or discomfort, stop the stretch immediately.
- Keep your movements slow and controlled.

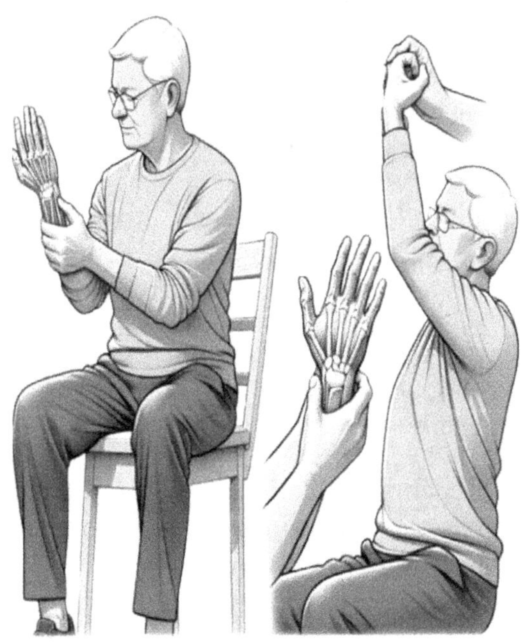

24. Shoulder Blade Pinches

Objective: Strengthens the muscles around the shoulder blades to improve posture.

Benefits:

- ✓ Enhances upper back strength, supporting better posture.
- ✓ Reduces the risk of shoulder and neck pain by promoting muscular balance.
- ✓ Improves shoulder blade mobility and stability.
- ✓ Aids in the prevention of rounded shoulders.

Steps:

1. Sit Upright: Sit on the edge of a chair with your feet flat on the ground and your spine straight. Relax your arms by your sides.

2. Pinch Shoulder Blades: Imagine there is a pencil between your shoulder blades. Pinch your shoulder blades together as if trying to hold the pencil in place, without shrugging your shoulders up.

3. Hold and Release: Hold the pinch for 5 seconds, then gently release and relax your shoulders.

4. Repetitions: Perform 10-15 repetitions, focusing on the movement of your shoulder blades and keeping the rest of your body relaxed.

5. Breathing: Breathe normally throughout the exercise, exhaling as you pinch the shoulder blades and inhaling as you release.

Safety Tips:

- Ensure movements are slow and controlled; avoid any jerky motions.
- Keep your neck relaxed and avoid shrugging your shoulders towards your ears.
- If you experience any discomfort, especially in the shoulders or back, reduce the intensity or take a break.

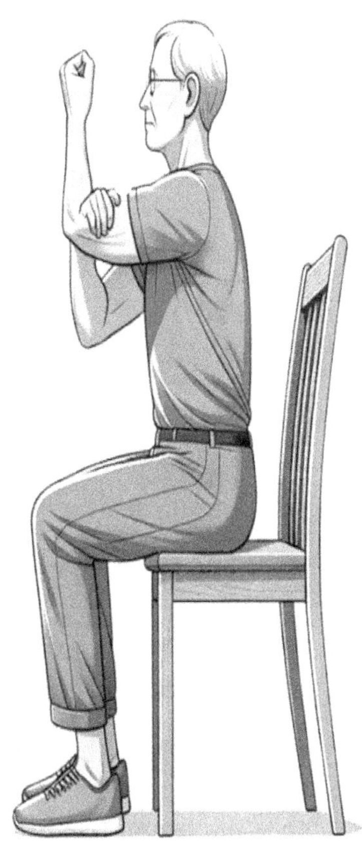

25. Seated Side Bends

Objective: Enhances lateral flexibility and strengthens the muscles along the sides of the torso.

Benefits:

- ✓ Increases flexibility and range of motion in the lateral (side) muscles of the torso.
- ✓ Helps relieve tension and stiffness in the side body, improving overall posture and alignment.
- ✓ Strengthens oblique muscles, contributing to core stability.
- ✓ Promotes better breathing by opening up the ribcage.

Steps:

1. Sit Upright: Sit on the edge of a chair with your feet flat on the ground, keeping your spine straight and tall. Place your hands on your hips or let them hang by your sides.

2. Perform the Side Bend: Slowly bend to the right, sliding your right hand down your leg towards the floor. Keep your left arm either on your hip, extended overhead, or hanging by your side, depending on your comfort and balance.

3. Hold the Stretch: Hold the side bend for 15-30 seconds, feeling a stretch along the left side of your torso. Keep your hips and shoulders facing forward, avoiding any forward or backward twisting.

4. Return to Center: Gently return to your starting upright position.
5. Repeat on the Other Side: Perform the same movement to the left side, focusing on stretching the right side of your body.
6. Repetitions: Aim for 2-3 repetitions on each side, or as needed for a good stretch.

Safety Tips:

- Move into and out of the bend slowly and with control to avoid any sudden movements.
- Keep your movements within a comfortable range to prevent overstretching.
- If you experience any discomfort or pain, especially in the back or hips, reduce the intensity of the stretch or skip the exercise.

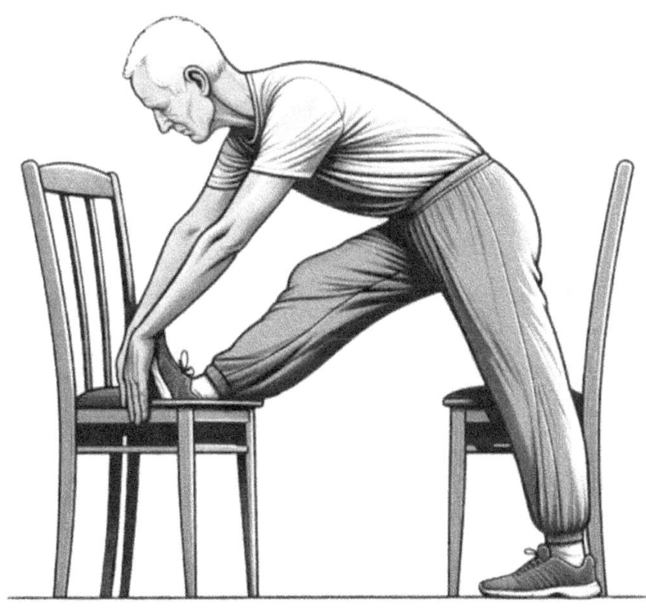

26. Seated Hamstring Stretch

Objective: To stretch the back of the thighs, improving flexibility and mobility in the hamstrings.

Benefits:

- ✓ Relieves tightness in the hamstrings, reducing the risk of lower back pain.
- ✓ Improves leg flexibility, aiding in mobility and daily activities.
- ✓ Enhances circulation in the legs.
- ✓ Can help prevent injuries related to muscle stiffness and imbalance.

Steps:

1. Sit Forward: Sit on the edge of a chair with your feet flat on the ground. Extend one leg straight in front of you, heel on the ground, and toes pointed up.

2. Maintain Posture: Keep your back straight and tall. Place your hands on the thigh of your bent leg for support.

3. Lean Forward: Slowly lean forward from your hips towards the extended leg. Keep your back straight and aim to bring your chest towards your knee. Feel the stretch along the back of your thigh.

4. Hold the Stretch: Hold the position for 15-30 seconds, breathing deeply and allowing the hamstring to gently stretch.

5. Switch Legs: Return to the starting position and repeat the stretch with the other leg extended.

6. Repetitions: Perform 2-3 repetitions on each leg, or as needed for a good stretch.

Safety Tips:

- Avoid rounding your back as you lean forward to prevent strain.
- If you feel any sharp pain or discomfort, ease up on the stretch.
- Keep the movements slow and controlled, focusing on feeling a gentle stretch in the hamstring.

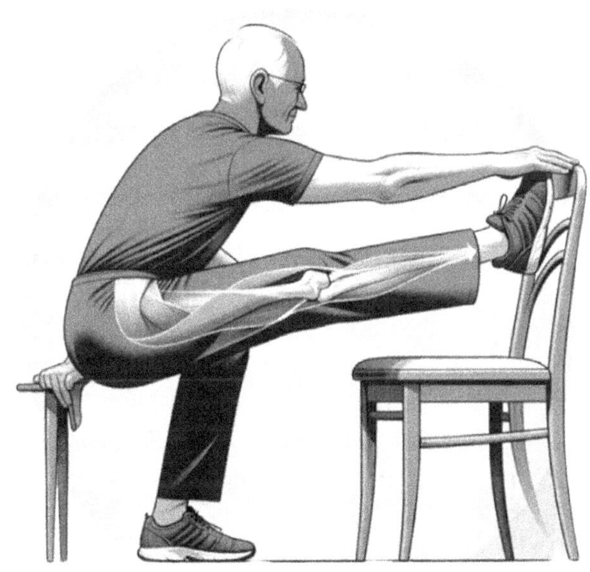

27. Calf Stretches

Objective: To relieve tightness in the calf muscles and improve ankle flexibility.

Benefits:

- ✓ Reduces the risk of calf muscle strains and injuries.
- ✓ Enhances flexibility in the lower legs, aiding in activities that require walking or climbing.
- ✓ Improves blood circulation in the legs.
- ✓ Helps prevent discomfort from conditions like plantar fasciitis.

Steps:

1. Sit Comfortably: Sit on a chair with your feet flat on the ground. Extend one leg out in front of you with the heel on the ground and the toes pointed upwards towards your shin.

2. Lean Forward: Keeping your back straight, lean forward slightly from your hips towards the extended leg. You should feel a stretch in the calf muscle of the extended leg.

3. Hold the Stretch: Hold this position for 15-30 seconds, focusing on a gentle stretch in the calf muscle. Avoid bouncing or forcing the stretch.

4. Switch Legs: Return to the starting position and repeat the stretch with the other leg.

5. Repetitions:Aim for 2-3 repetitions on each leg, or as needed to feel a good stretch.

Safety Tips:

- Ensure your movements are slow and controlled to avoid overstretching.
- Keep your back straight to prevent strain as you lean forward.
- If you experience any sharp pain, stop the stretch immediately.

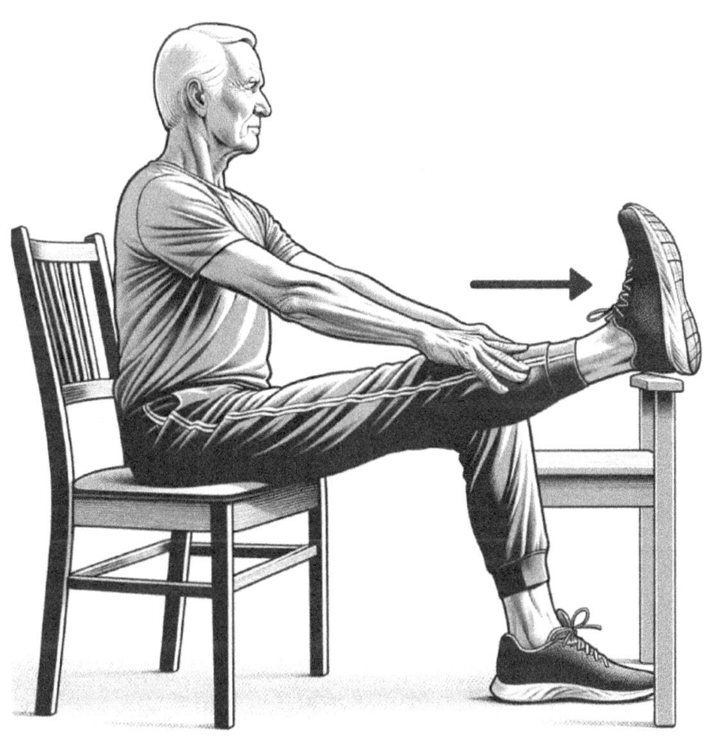

28. Seated Figure Four Stretch

Objective: To open the hips and stretch the glutes and piriformis muscle.

Benefits:

- ✓ Relieves tightness and discomfort in the hips and lower back.
- ✓ Improves hip mobility and flexibility.
- ✓ Can help alleviate symptoms of sciatica.
- ✓ Enhances overall posture by promoting hip alignment.

Steps:

1. Start Seated: Sit on the edge of a chair with your feet flat on the ground, hip-width apart.

2. Position Your Leg: Lift your right foot off the ground and place your right ankle on your left thigh, just above the knee. Allow your right knee to drop open to the side.

3. Increase the Stretch: Gently lean forward from your hips, keeping your back straight. You should feel a stretch in your right hip and glute.

4. Hold the Stretch: Maintain this position for 15-30 seconds, breathing deeply and focusing on relaxing into the stretch.

5. Switch Sides: Carefully return to the starting position and repeat the stretch with your left foot on your right thigh.

6. Repetitions: Aim for 2-3 repetitions on each side, adjusting as needed for comfort and flexibility.

- Perform the stretch gently to avoid putting undue pressure on your knee.
- Keep your foot flexed during the stretch to stabilize the ankle and protect the knee joint.
- If you experience any sharp pain or discomfort, especially in the knee, adjust your position or discontinue the stretch.

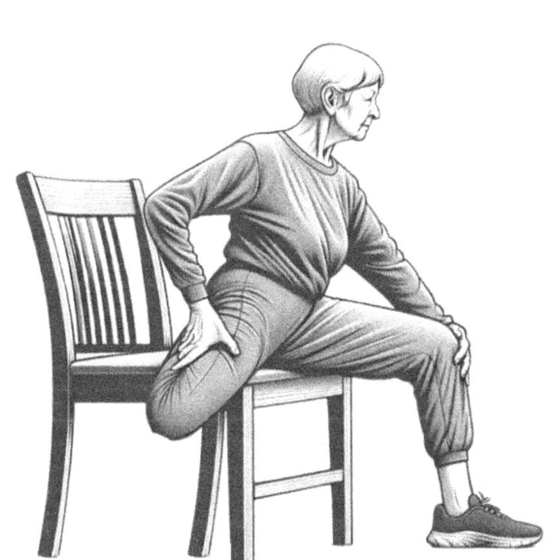

29. Neck Rotations

Objective: Increases mobility and relieves tension in the neck.

Benefits:

- ✓ Enhances neck flexibility and range of motion.
- ✓ Relieves stiffness and tension in the neck and upper shoulders.
- ✓ Can help reduce headaches and improve posture.
- ✓ Promotes relaxation and stress relief.
- ✓

Steps:

1. Sit Comfortably: Begin seated on a chair with your feet flat on the ground, spine straight, and shoulders relaxed.

2. Start Rotation: Slowly turn your head to the right, aiming to look over your right shoulder. Keep your shoulders still and facing forward.

3. Hold and Return: Hold the position for a few seconds, feeling a gentle stretch along the left side of your neck. Return your head to the center.

4. Repeat on the Left: Turn your head to the left, looking over your left shoulder, and hold for a few seconds to stretch the right side of your neck.

5. Full Rotation: If comfortable, gently rotate your head in a full circle, starting from one shoulder, dropping the chin to the chest, moving to the other shoulder, and tilting the head back. Perform this movement slowly and only within a comfortable range of motion.

6. Repetitions:** Perform 3-5 rotations in each direction, focusing on smooth, controlled movements.

Safety Tips:

- Move your head slowly and gently to avoid dizziness or strain.
- Do not force your head beyond its comfortable range of motion.
- If you experience any pain or discomfort, especially in the neck or upper back, reduce the range of motion or discontinue the exercise.

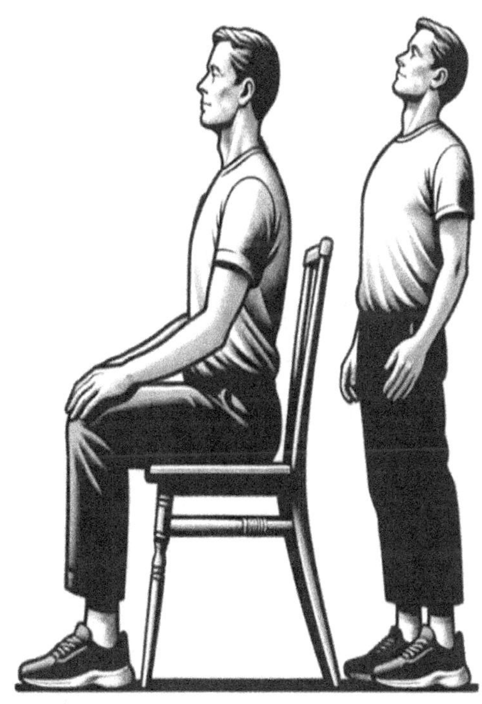

30. Seated Ankle Flexion and Extension

Objective: Strengthens the ankles and improves flexibility.

Benefits:

- ✓ Enhances the range of motion and flexibility in the ankle joints.
- ✓ Promotes better circulation in the lower legs and feet.
- ✓ Reduces the risk of ankle stiffness and injuries.
- ✓ Supports overall foot health and mobility.

Steps:

1.Sit Comfortably: Begin by sitting on a chair with your feet flat on the ground, spine straight, and shoulders relaxed.

2. Extend One Leg: Extend one leg out in front of you, keeping the leg slightly lifted so that your foot is not touching the ground.

3. Flex and Extend the Ankle:

- Flexion: Point your toes upward, bringing them towards your shin to stretch the calf muscles.
- Extension: Point your toes downward, stretching the front of your ankle and shin.

4. Alternate Movements: Continue alternating between flexion and extension, focusing on a full range of motion in the ankle joint.

5. Switch Legs: After completing a set of 10-15 repetitions, switch to the other leg and repeat the exercise.

6. Repetitions: Aim for 2-3 sets per leg, or as comfortable.

Safety Tips:

- Perform the movements slowly and with control to avoid jerking the ankle.
- If you experience any pain or discomfort in the ankle, reduce the range of motion or stop the exercise.
- Ensure you're seated securely on the chair to avoid slipping.

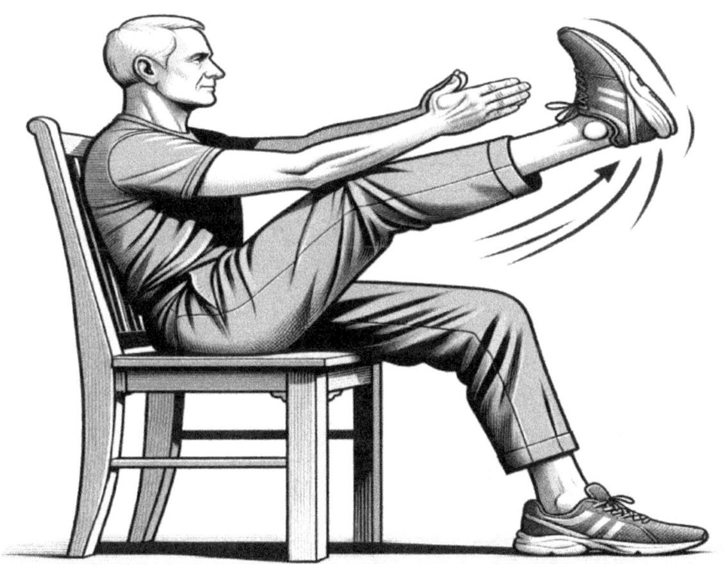

31. Upper Back and Shoulder Stretch

Objective: Utilizes a towel or a strap to provide a deep stretch across the shoulders and upper back.

Benefits:

- ✓ Relieves tension and stiffness in the shoulders and upper back.
- ✓ Enhances flexibility and range of motion in the shoulder joints.
- ✓ Promotes better posture by opening up the chest and shoulders.
- ✓ Can alleviate pain associated with poor posture or prolonged sitting.

Steps:

1. Sit Upright: Sit on a chair with your feet flat on the ground and your spine straight.

2. Hold the Towel/Strap: Hold a towel or strap with both hands, wider than shoulder-width apart. Extend your arms in front of you at shoulder height.

3. Lift Your Arms: Keeping your grip on the towel/strap, slowly lift your arms overhead, keeping them as straight as possible.

6. Stretch Your Back: Gently pull on the towel/strap as you lift, feeling the stretch across your shoulders and upper back. If comfortable, slightly arch your back to deepen the stretch.

5. Hold and Return: Hold the position for 15-30 seconds, then carefully lower your arms back to the starting position.

6. Repetitions: Perform 2-3 repetitions, focusing on a deep stretch with each lift.

Safety Tips:

- Keep the movements slow and controlled to avoid overstretching.
- Adjust the width of your grip on the towel/strap to suit your flexibility.
- Breathe deeply throughout the stretch to enhance relaxation and effectiveness.

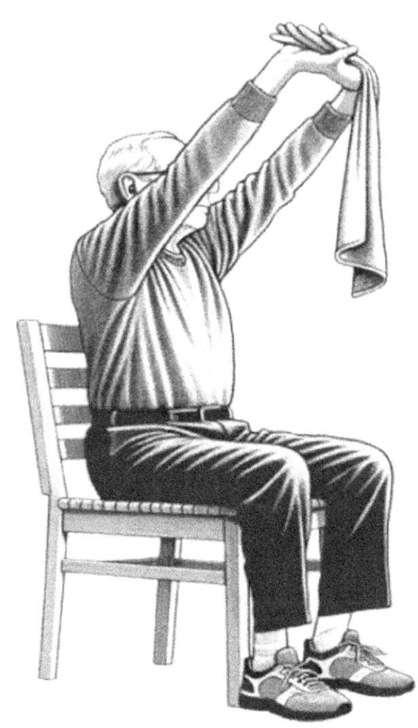

32. Toe Spread and Squeeze

Objective: To improve toe mobility and strength, enhancing balance and foot health.

Benefits:

- ✓ Increases flexibility and range of motion in the toes.
- ✓ Strengthens foot muscles, contributing to better balance and stability.
- ✓ Helps prevent foot problems related to tightness and immobility, such as bunions and hammertoes.
- ✓ Promotes circulation in the feet, which can be beneficial for those with conditions like diabetes or peripheral neuropathy.

Steps:

1. Sit Comfortably: Begin seated on a chair with your feet flat on the ground and your spine straight.

2. Focus on Your Toes: Lift one foot off the ground slightly. Spread your toes as wide as you can, holding the spread for a few seconds.

3. Squeeze Your Toes: After spreading your toes, try to squeeze them together or curl them inward, holding this position for a few seconds as well.

4. Alternate Movements: Continue alternating between spreading and squeezing your toes for several repetitions.

5. Switch Feet: After completing a set of repetitions on one foot, place it back on the ground and repeat the exercise with your other foot.

6. Repetitions: Aim for 10-15 repetitions of spreading and squeezing on each foot, or as comfortable.

Safety Tips:

- Perform the exercises gently to avoid cramping. If you experience cramps, pause and gently massage your foot.
- If you have any foot conditions or injuries, consult with a healthcare provider before starting this exercise.
- Ensure you're seated securely on the chair to maintain balance while lifting one foot.

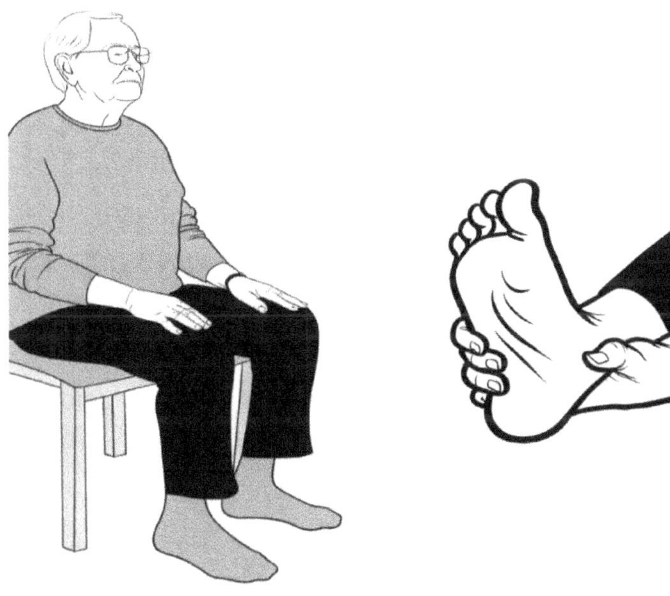

33. Seated Hip Circles

Objective: Mobilizes the hip joint and strengthens the hip muscles.

Benefits:

- ✓ Improves hip mobility and flexibility.
- ✓ Enhances circulation in the hip area, which can reduce stiffness and discomfort.
- ✓ Strengthens muscles around the hips, contributing to better stability and balance.
- ✓ Can alleviate lower back pain by promoting better hip alignment and movement.

Steps:

1. Start in a Seated Position: Sit on the edge of a chair with your feet flat on the ground and your spine straight. Place your hands on your hips or the sides of the chair for stability.

2. Initiate the Circles: Shift your hips to the right, then gently move them back, to the left, and finally forward, creating a circular motion. Imagine drawing a circle with your hips.

3. Keep the Movement Controlled:** Focus on smooth, controlled movements, keeping the upper body as still as possible to isolate the motion in the hips.

4. Change Directions: After completing 5-10 circles in one direction, reverse the direction of your hip circles, ensuring an even stretch and strengthening on both sides.

5. Repetitions: Aim for 2-3 sets of circles in each direction, or as comfortable.

Safety Tips:

- Move slowly and within a comfortable range of motion to avoid straining the hips or lower back.
- If you experience any pain, especially in the hips or lower back, reduce the range of motion or stop the exercise.
- Ensure the chair is stable and won't move during the exercise.

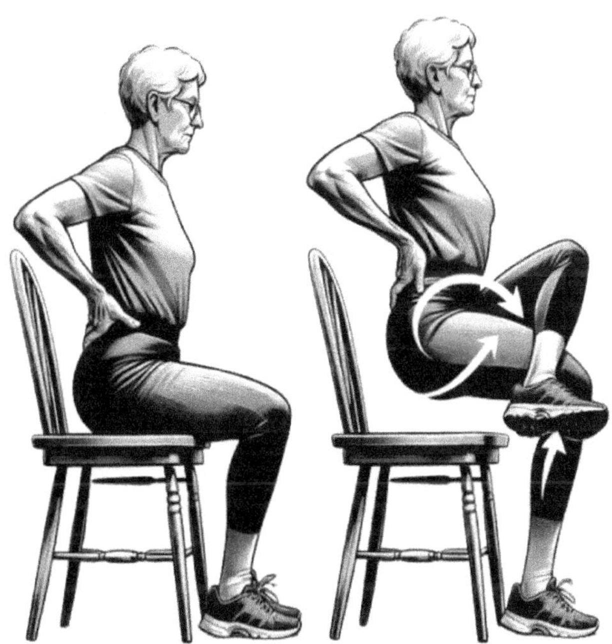

34. Elbow Circles

Objective: Enhances elbow joint mobility and flexibility.

Benefits:

- ✓ Improves range of motion and flexibility in the elbow joints.
- ✓ Helps reduce stiffness and discomfort in the arms and forearms.
- ✓ Promotes better circulation and muscle engagement around the elbow area.
- ✓ Supports overall arm health and functionality.

Steps:

1. Sit Comfortably: Begin by sitting on a chair with your feet flat on the ground and your spine straight. Let your arms hang loosely by your sides.

2. Bend Your Elbows: Lift your arms and bend your elbows so your forearms are parallel to the ground, and your hands are pointing upwards.

3. Perform the Circles: Slowly rotate your elbows in small circles, focusing on moving only the lower part of your arms. Keep your shoulders and upper arms as still as possible.

4. Change Directions: After completing 10-15 circles in one direction, reverse and perform the circles in the opposite direction.

5. Repetitions: Aim for 2-3 sets of circles in each direction, adjusting as needed based on comfort and flexibility.

Safety Tips:

Safety Tips:

- Keep the movements slow and controlled to avoid any strain on the elbow joints.
- If you experience any pain or discomfort in the elbows, reduce the size of the circles or stop the exercise.
- Ensure you're seated securely on the chair to maintain balance throughout the exercise.

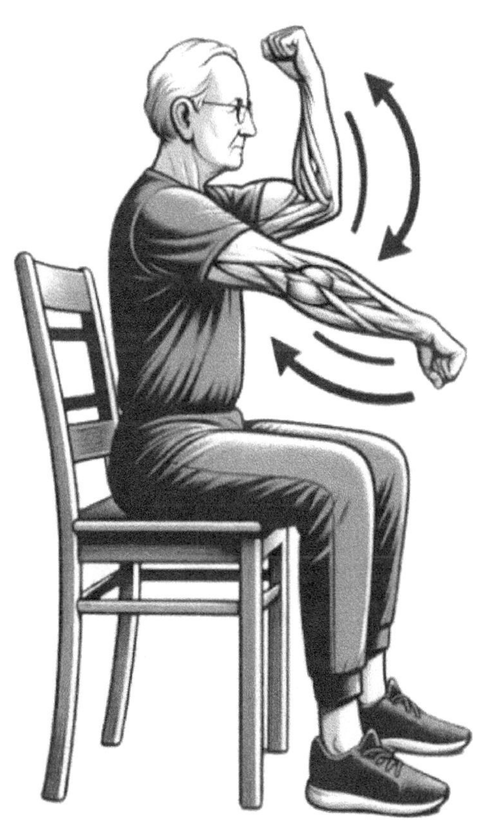

35. Seated Torso Twists

Objective: To engage the core muscles and further mobilize the spine with a gentle twist.

Benefits:

- ✓ Increases spinal flexibility and range of motion.
- ✓ Engages and strengthens the core muscles, including the obliques.
- ✓ Can help alleviate lower back stiffness and improve posture.
- ✓ Promotes digestion and abdominal organ health through gentle compression.

Steps:

1. Sit Upright: Begin by sitting on the edge of a chair with your feet flat on the ground, spine straight, and arms relaxed by your sides.

2. Initiate the Twist: Extend your arms out in front of you at shoulder height. Slowly twist your torso to the right, keeping your hips facing forward. You can place your left hand on your right knee and your right hand on the chair behind you to deepen the twist.

3. Hold the Twist: Hold the position for a few seconds, focusing on stretching the spine and engaging your core muscles.

4. Return to Center: Slowly untwist your torso, bringing your arms back in front of you.

5. Repeat on the Other Side: Perform the twist to the left side, using the opposite hands for support.

6. Repetitions: Aim for 5-10 repetitions on each side, or as comfortable, focusing on smooth, controlled movements.

Safety Tips:

- Move into and out of the twist slowly to avoid dizziness or strain.
- Keep the twist gentle, especially if you have any spinal conditions or discomfort.
- Ensure the chair is stable and won't move during the exercise.

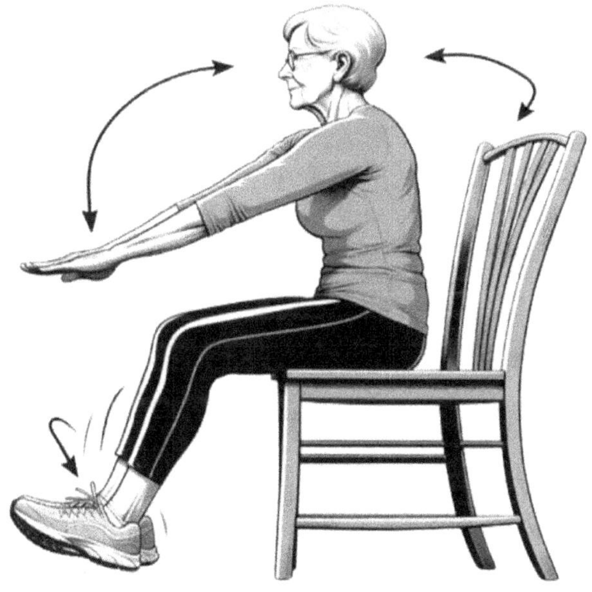

36. Chair Push-Ups

Objective: Strengthen the arms and chest using the chair for support.

Benefits:

- ✓ Enhances upper body strength, particularly in the arms, chest, and shoulders.
- ✓ Improves stability and muscle endurance.
- ✓ Can aid in maintaining joint mobility and reducing the risk of upper body strain.
- ✓ Supports activities that require pushing movements.

Steps:

1. Position Your Chair: Ensure your chair is stable and up against a wall to prevent it from moving.

2. Start in the Initial Position: Stand facing the chair, place your hands on the seat's edge slightly wider than shoulder-width apart.

3. Lower Your Body: Bend your elbows to lower your body towards the chair while keeping your feet flat on the ground. Your body should form a straight line from your head to your heels.

4. Push Up: Push through your hands to return to the starting position, extending your arms fully.

5. Repetitions: Aim for 8-12 push-ups, or as many as you can perform with good form. Consider doing 2-3 sets.

Safety Tips:

- Make sure the chair is securely placed against a wall or a stable surface to prevent slipping.
- Keep your core engaged throughout the exercise to support your lower back.
- Adjust the difficulty by stepping closer or further away from the chair, affecting the angle of your push-up.

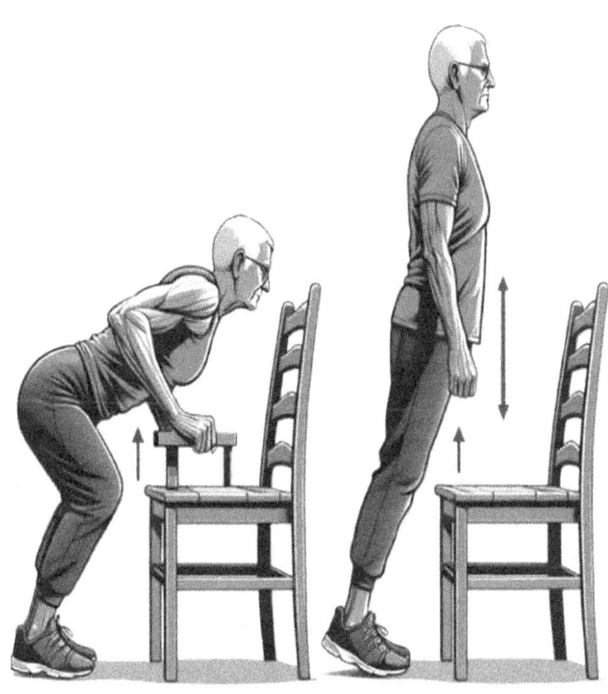

17. Seated Knee Extensions

Objective: Strengthens the quadriceps and improves knee joint stability.

Benefits:

- ✓ Enhances strength in the quadriceps, which are crucial for walking, standing, and maintaining balance.
- ✓ Supports knee health by improving joint stability and flexibility.
- ✓ Can aid in reducing knee pain and stiffness.
- ✓ Promotes better circulation in the legs.

Steps:

1. Sit Upright: Begin by sitting on a chair with your feet flat on the ground, spine straight, and hands resting on the sides of the chair or on your lap.

2. Extend One Leg: Slowly extend one leg out in front of you, aiming to straighten the knee as much as possible. Keep your foot flexed, toes pointing upwards.

3. Hold and Lower: Hold the extended position for a few seconds, focusing on contracting the quadriceps muscles, then slowly lower your foot back to the ground.

4. Switch Legs: Repeat the exercise with your other leg.

5. Repetitions: Aim for 10-15 repetitions on each leg, or as comfortable. Consider performing 2-3 sets for a more comprehensive workout.

Safety Tips:

+ Ensure the chair is stable and will not move during the exercise.
+ Keep your movements slow and controlled to maximize muscle engagement and prevent jerky motions.
+ If you experience any discomfort or pain, especially in the knees, adjust the intensity or consult with a healthcare provider.

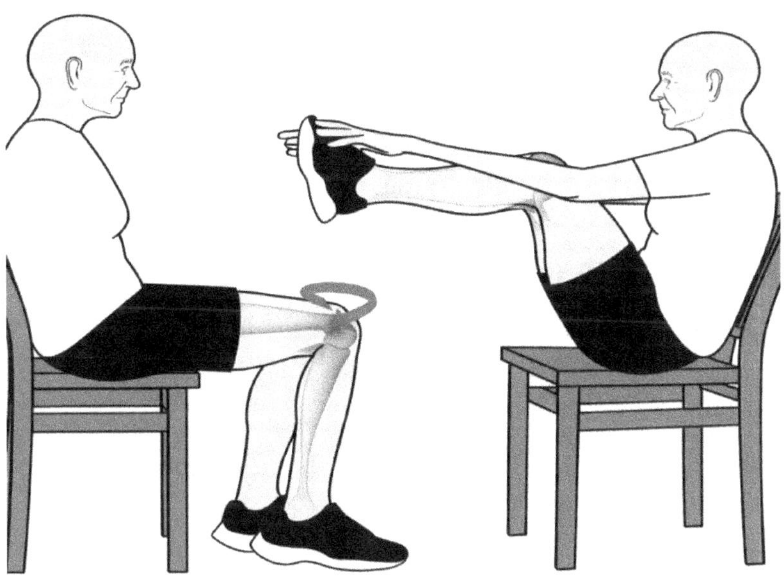

38. Hand Clench and Release

Objective: To improve hand strength and flexibility, beneficial for arthritis relief and maintaining fine motor skills.

Benefits:

- ✓ Enhances grip strength and dexterity.
- ✓ Promotes flexibility in the fingers and hand joints.
- ✓ Can help alleviate stiffness and pain associated with conditions like arthritis.
- ✓ Supports daily activities that require hand strength, such as opening jars or writing.

Steps:

1. Start Seated: Sit comfortably on a chair with your feet flat on the ground and your spine straight. Relax your arms by your sides or place them on your lap.

2. Clench Your Hands: Slowly clench your fists, squeezing your hands as tightly as comfortable. Focus on engaging the muscles in your fingers and palms.

3. Hold and Release: Hold the clenched position for a few seconds, then slowly release, spreading your fingers wide apart.

4. Repeat: Continue alternating between clenching and releasing your hands for several repetitions.

5. Repetitions: Aim for 10-15 repetitions, or as many as comfortable, focusing on smooth, controlled movements.

- Perform the exercise gently to avoid overstraining your hand muscles.
- If you experience any sharp pain or discomfort, especially in the joints, reduce the intensity or stop the exercise.
- Breathe normally throughout the exercise to promote relaxation and enhance the benefits.

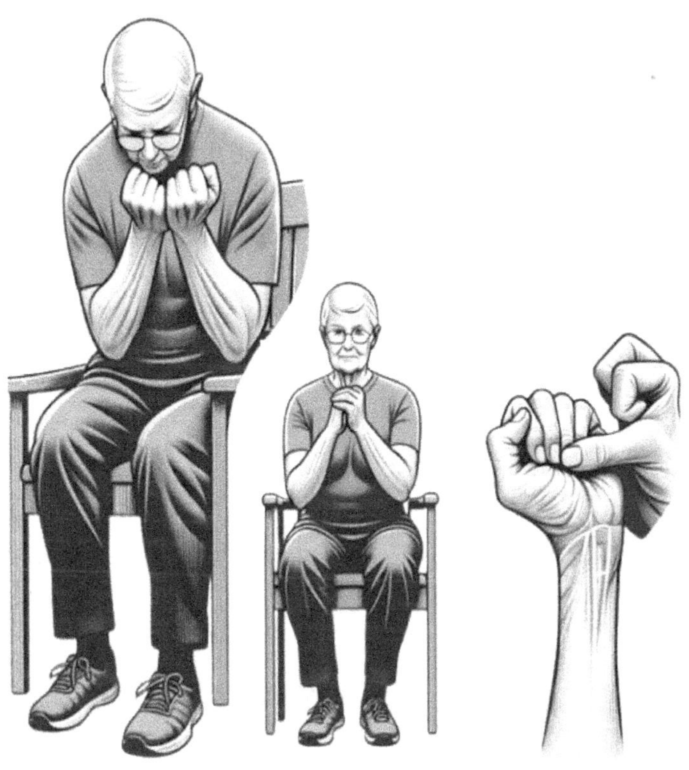

39. Seated Calf Raises

Objective: Strengthens the lower legs and improves ankle stability.

Benefits:

- ✓ Enhances strength in the calf muscles, important for walking and climbing stairs.
- ✓ Supports ankle stability and flexibility.
- ✓ Promotes circulation in the lower legs, which can reduce swelling and prevent venous issues.
- ✓ Can aid in balancing and preventing falls by strengthening the lower body.

Steps:

1. Start Seated: Sit on a chair with your feet flat on the ground, hip-width apart, and your spine straight.

2. Perform the Calf Raise: Press down through the balls of your feet to lift your heels as high off the ground as you comfortably can, engaging your calf muscles.

3. Hold and Lower: Hold the raised position for a moment, feeling the contraction in your calf muscles, then slowly lower your heels back to the ground.

4. Repetitions: Aim for 10-15 repetitions, or as many as comfortable, focusing on controlled movements.

5. Sets: Consider performing 2-3 sets for a more comprehensive lower leg workout.

- Ensure the chair is stable and won't move during the exercise.
- Move slowly and with control to maximize muscle engagement and prevent any jerky movements.
- If you experience any discomfort or pain, especially in the ankles or calves, adjust the intensity or consult with a healthcare provider.

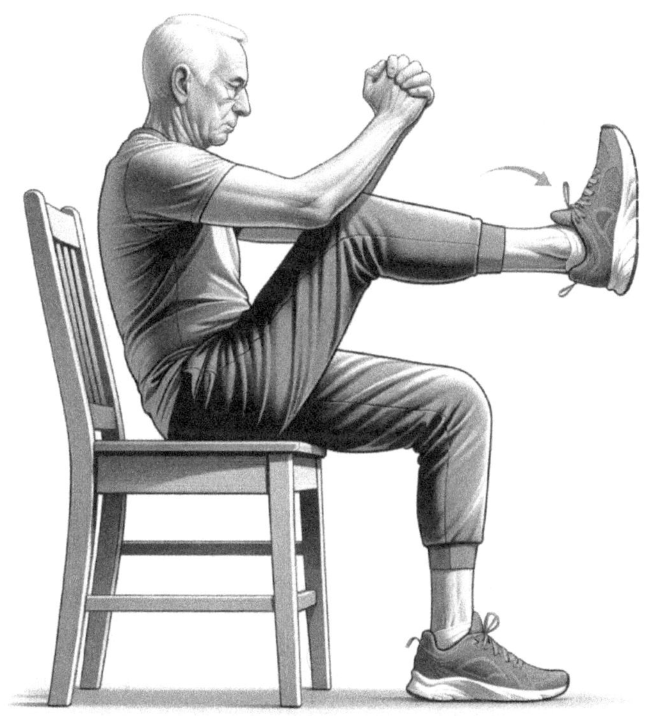

40. Breathing Exercises

Objective: Focuses on deep, diaphragmatic breathing to enhance relaxation and lung capacity.

Benefits:

- ✓ Improves oxygenation of the body, supporting overall health and well-being.
- ✓ Promotes relaxation and stress relief, reducing anxiety and promoting a calm mind.
- ✓ Enhances lung capacity and efficiency, beneficial for respiratory health.
- ✓ Can improve posture and core stability through the engagement of the diaphragm and abdominal muscles during deep breaths.

Steps:

1. Find a Comfortable Seat: Sit comfortably on a chair with your feet flat on the ground, spine straight, and shoulders relaxed.

2.Place Your Hands: Place one hand on your chest and the other on your abdomen to feel the movement of your breath.

3.Inhale Deeply: Slowly inhale through your nose, allowing your abdomen to expand fully, feeling the hand on it rise. The hand on your chest should move very little.

4. Exhale Slowly: Exhale through your mouth, gently contracting your abdominal muscles to help push the air out, feeling the hand on your abdomen lower.

5. Continue Breathing: Repeat this deep breathing pattern for several minutes, focusing on slow, controlled breaths that fill and empty your lungs completely.

6. Practice Regularly: Aim to incorporate these breathing exercises into your daily routine, especially during moments of stress or when you need to relax.

- If you feel dizzy or lightheaded at any point, pause and return to normal breathing.
- Ensure you are in a comfortable position that allows for unobstructed breathing.
- These exercises can be performed multiple times a day to promote relaxation and improve breathing.

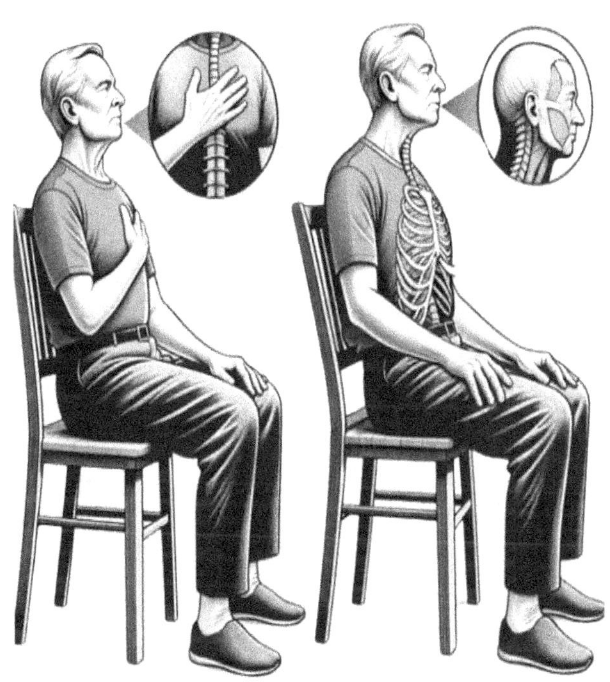

21 Days - challenge

Week 1: Foundation and Flexibility

- ❖ Day 1: Introduction to Deep Breathing Exercises. Practice for 10 minutes.
- ❖ Day 2: Seated Calf Raises (15 repetitions × 2 sets) + Seated Ankle Flexion and Extension (10 repetitions per foot).
- ❖ Day 3: Seated Hamstring Stretch (30 seconds per leg × 2) + Seated Figure Four Stretch (30 seconds per side).
- ❖ Day 4: Shoulder Blade Pinches (10 repetitions × 2 sets) + Upper Back and Shoulder Stretch with a towel (30 seconds × 2).
- ❖ Day 5: Wrist Flexor and Extensor Stretches (30 seconds per stretch per arm) + Hand Clench and Release (15 repetitions).
- ❖ Day 6: Seated Side Bends (10 repetitions per side) + Seated Torso Twists (10 repetitions per side).
- ❖ Day 7: Reflection and Deep Breathing. Reflect on the week's progress and engage in a 15-minute deep breathing session.

Week 2: Strength and Stability

- ❖ Day 8: Chair Push-Ups (8-12 repetitions × 2 sets) + Seated Knee Extensions (10 repetitions per leg × 2 sets).
- ❖ Day 9: Elbow Circles (10 circles per direction) + Seated "T" Pose (hold 30 seconds × 2).
- ❖ Day 10: Seated Bicycle Crunches (10 repetitions per side) + Seated Leg Lifts (10 repetitions per leg).

- ❖ Day 11: Toe Spread and Squeeze (15 repetitions per foot) + Seated Hip Circles (10 circles per direction).
- ❖ Day 12: Seated Knee Lifts with a Twist (10 repetitions per side) + Seated Calf Raises (15 repetitions × 2 sets).
- ❖ Day 13: Arm and Leg Lifts (10 repetitions per side) + Neck Rotations (5 rotations per direction).
- ❖ Day 14: Mid-challenge Reflection. Reflect on the past week and practice deep breathing for 15 minutes.

Week 3: Consolidation and Mindfulness

- ❖ Day 15: Combine any two flexibility exercises from Week 1.
- ❖ Day 16: Combine any two strength exercises from Week 2.
- ❖ Day 17: Choose any three exercises from Week 1 or Week 2 that you found most beneficial.
- ❖ Day 18: Deep Breathing and Meditation. Engage in a 20-minute session focusing on mindfulness and relaxation.
- ❖ Day 19: Create a personalized routine combining your favorite exercises from the challenge.

* Day 20: Practice your personalized routine.
* Day 21: Reflect on the 21-day challenge. Note any changes in your physical or mental well-being and plan how to incorporate these practices into your daily life.

This 21-day challenge is designed to gradually build a habit of regular physical activity and mindfulness practice. Feel free to adjust the exercises and durations to suit your fitness level and preferences.

Conclusion

In our journey through " Chair Yoga Revolution for Seniors Over 60," we've explored accessible yet powerful practices designed to enhance your physical strength, flexibility, and inner calm. From the very first day, we embarked on a path not just to reclaim, but to redefine what our bodies can achieve in our later years. Each pose, each breath, and each moment of stillness was a step towards greater balance, mobility, and a deeper sense of peace within ourselves.

As we conclude this 21-day challenge, remember that the end of this guide is not the end of your journey. The practices you've learned are tools for life—meant to be revisited, refined, and integrated into your daily routine. The improvements in balance, strength, mobility, and mental clarity you've begun to experience are just the beginning. With regular practice, these benefits will continue to grow, enhancing your quality of life and independence.

Beyond the physical benefits, I hope you've discovered a deeper connection to yourself. Chair yoga is not just about the poses; it's a practice of mindfulness, a way to tune into your body's needs and honor them. It's a reminder that age is but a number, and that our spirits can remain vibrant and youthful even as we navigate the challenges of aging.

As you move forward, I encourage you to keep exploring what your body is capable of with an open heart and mind. Let the principles of chair yoga guide you—not just on the mat, but in every aspect of life. Approach each day with the same intention and presence you bring to your practice, and watch the transformation unfold.

Thank you for allowing me to be a part of your journey. May you continue to grow stronger, more flexible, and more centered with each passing day. Remember, the true power of chair yoga lies not in achieving the perfect pose, but in the practice itself—in the courage to start, the perseverance to continue, and the openness to experience whatever comes your way.

Namaste.

As we wrap up our journey with " Chair Yoga Revolution for Seniors Over 60," I hope you've found value and growth through its pages. If this guide has positively impacted your life, please consider leaving a review. Your feedback is not only deeply appreciated but also helps others on similar paths discover the benefits of chair yoga. A few words about your experience can make a significant difference. Thank you for your support and for being part of this wellness journey.

Warmest regards,

[Clara Harper]

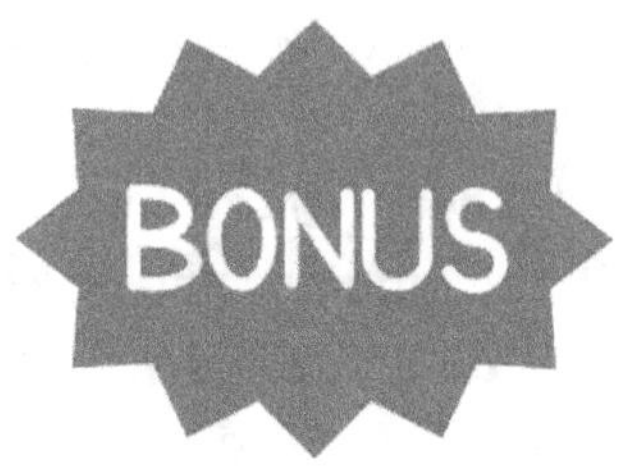

Click the link to get your bonus or scan the QR code

BONUS ONE FREE PRINTABLE JOURNAL

Click here to get your bonus